PRESCRIPTION FOR DISASTER

THE HIDDEN DANGERS IN YOUR MEDICINE CABINET

Thomas J. Moore

A DELL BOOK

Published by
Dell Publishing
a division of
Random House, Inc.
1540 Broadway
New York, New York 10036

ISBN: 0-440-23484-0

Reprinted by arrangement with Simon & Schuster

Printed in the United States of America

Published simultaneously in Canada

February 1999

10 9 8 7 6 5 4 3 2 1
WCD

GET A DOSE OF REALITY!
FIND OUT . . .

- When Tylenol, Aleve, or Motrin can send you to the hospital
- Why antibiotics can be deadly
- How Prozac and Zoloft can affect your sex life
- Which recently approved drugs caused cancer in animals
- What important warning comes with America's best-selling blood pressure drug
- Which sleep medication put the head of the Supreme Court in detox?
- How you can get all the facts you need . . .
  . . . and more!

ALSO BY
THOMAS J. MOORE

Deadly Medicine

Lifespan

Heart Failure

**IN MEMORY OF
THEODORE A. HUNT**

WARNING

In ethics and in law, the final decision about any medical therapy, including whether to take a prescription drug, belongs solely to the patient.

Nevertheless, readers of this book are strongly urged to seek medical advice before stopping or altering the dose of a drug outside the range in the prescribing information.

Stopping some drugs abruptly may cause sudden rebound or withdrawal effects. If multiple drugs are being taken, stopping one drug can sometimes change the effect of another.

A section of this book will describe the steps you can take should you become concerned about the drugs you are now taking.

CONTENTS

PART ONE

THE NATURE OF DRUGS

CHAPTER ONE

Warning Flags

AMY AND GARY KAUFMAN were vacationing in the British Virgin Islands at the lovely resort at Little Dix Bay. Their young children were at home in Atlanta. They had spent an idyllic day, sailing and swimming in the crystal-clear Caribbean Sea. For dinner they joined two friends. Amy had a Caesar salad and lobster in a puff pastry, and two glasses of wine.

As they got ready for bed, Amy had a question. Several months earlier, she had seen a dermatologist for an outbreak of hives. She came home with a prescription for a popular nonsedating antihistamine called Hismanal. As instructed, she took one tablet every morning. But that evening after dinner, her hives still bothered her. Could she take an extra tablet at bedtime? Gary Kaufman will never forget his answer. Since Kaufman is a neurosurgeon, Amy was asking a medical doctor as well as her husband. "One tablet can't kill you," he said. After she took the extra tablet, they went to bed.

When Kaufman awoke the next morning, his wife was dead.

She was still lying beside him in bed. But her body was cooling to room temperature, and her hands and feet were already stiffening with rigor mortis. He shipped her refrigerated body back to the United States for autopsy. The report said Amy's death was caused by cardiac arrest and implicated Hismanal.[1] The whole episode was so traumatic for Gary Kaufman that he abandoned the practice of medicine.

From the beginning, Hismanal was a leading suspect. The manufacturer had reported that cardiac arrests had been observed with as little as one extra tablet.[2] In 1997, the FDA proposed to withdraw a very similar drug, Seldane, on safety grounds but inexplicably took no action on a drug with comparable risks.[3] By May 1994, Hismanal had been linked to at least eighty-two cases of erratic heart rhythms so dangerous they required hospitalization even at the recommended dose of one tablet.[4]

If Gary and Amy Kaufman had been in a minor auto accident on a Sunday drive, the authorities would have become involved immediately. In most states, even $150 in minor damage would bring a paid public servant—a police officer—to take a detailed report. Such reports would be analyzed for lessons about automobile safety. Almost any other kind of accident that results in death typically receives intense official scrutiny. A lethal fire, boating accident, or commercial airplane crash brings trained investigators to the site immediately. But when a prescription drug is suspected of killing a person, the health professionals on the scene have no obligation to file a report about the drug—and rarely do so.[5] But how serious are the dangers of drugs? How many times every year does a tragedy strike?

One place to check is the death statistics. The nation's official death count is kept by a small federal agency called the National Center for Health Statistics. Each year, it collects data from every single death certificate—in 1995 the total was

2,312,132 deaths.[6] Among the seventy-two listed major causes of death, no entry can be found for deaths caused by prescription drugs. However, the major causes of death did include the 6 deaths caused by whooping cough and the 277 women who died in childbirth. Each year a few hundred certificates may indicate a drug overdose or poisoning by drugs. But in most cases where prescription drugs were likely responsible, the cause of death will be listed as something else, perhaps cardiac arrest, infection, internal bleeding, or liver disease. In a chain of failure beginning with the attending physicians and ending at the center's computer data files, the system is simply not set up to monitor this important threat to public health.

Another obvious candidate for monitoring the overall hazards of prescription drugs is the Food and Drug Administration. It operates an adverse reaction reporting system with a catchy name—MedWatch—but with shortcomings that are embarrassing. It is entirely voluntary and routinely shunned by most physicians. In an article in the *Journal of the American Medical Association*, then FDA Commissioner David A. Kessler revealed that "only about 1% of serious events are reported to the FDA."[7] Although the FDA had just completed a program to make it easier for doctors to report serious events, the agency believed the real obstacle was the prevailing attitudes among American doctors. "It is not in the culture of U.S. medicine to notify the FDA about adverse events," Kessler noted. The first important warning flag is to discover a safety system in which no one even investigates or keeps an official count of the most serious accidents.

From the most senior public health officials to the daily consumers of medication, people just don't want to think about the risks of this inherently risky business. Doctors don't want to scare their patients or draw attention to their own prescribing mistakes. Serious safety questions about a major drug can threaten the survival of a large drug company. As a result, companies often wage aggressive campaigns against safety critics. Even the FDA has a dilemma. Every time it moves to restrict or withdraw a dangerous drug, it has to face questions about why it allowed the drug to reach the market in the first place.

Periodically, a major public official or health researcher surveys the woefully inadequate data and estimates the lives lost each year to prescription drugs. How many Amy Kaufmans die every year? Prescription drugs in medical use are involved in about 100,000 deaths a year.[8] This total is four times as many as die from homicide and more than double the death toll from auto accidents. Prescription drugs pose a major peril to public health.

As we shall see later, injury and disability are a much more common complication of prescription drugs than death. Over a lifetime of drug taking, the average American has a 26 percent chance of being hospitalized from a drug injury. Long-term use of just one class of drugs—anti-inflammatory agents such as aspirin, ibuprofen and Naprosyn—causes an estimated 70,000 hospitalizations every year.[9] In fact, prescription drugs are ten times more likely to put you in the hospital than an automobile accident. These estimates do not include the millions of people who suffer severe adverse reactions that do not require hospitalization but nevertheless cause major human suffering or permanent disability.

Not only are the risks of drugs studiously ignored, but American society seems eager to embrace their hoped-for benefits with a breathtaking lack of critical scrutiny. In the summer of 1995, the public learned about leptin, a new miracle drug for obesity.[10] Researchers had discovered that leptin was a human and animal hormone that helps regulate body fat. When given the missing protein, genetically obese mice shed 30 percent of their body weight in just a few weeks' time. Even normal mice lost 12 percent of their body fat after being fed leptin. The world gazed in wonder at pictures on the television news that showed the pudgy mice miraculously made svelte. As soon as they heard about leptin, people wanted it immediately. Phones were ringing off the hook at Amgen, the California biotech company that had used genetic-engineering technology to manufacture the natural hormone. One television reporter was so eager he was actually pleading with an Amgen spokesman to say how soon the drug would be available. The stories implied that testing in humans was a mere formality. One can almost imagine the coming attacks on the Food and Drug Administration for keeping people from getting this important new drug.

Blind faith in the wonders of medical science had reached dangerous levels when people were so eager for a new drug that had not yet been given to a single human being. This credulity extended to the highest levels of the medical research establishment. Phillip Gorden, the senior researcher on obesity at the National Institutes of Health, said in the *Washington Post*, "We have every reason to believe this could become a major treatment for obesity in humans. It should be effective independent of the cause of obesity, except maybe in certain rare cases."[11]

Within a matter of weeks, an elementary scientific experiment had crushed any immediate prospects for the wonder drug leptin. A Canadian medical researcher had determined the leptin levels in fourteen grossly obese subjects, and compared them to eleven lean people. The obese typically had leptin levels that were twenty to thirty times higher than the lean subjects.[12] This was not the missing hormone to regulate fat; the obese were loaded with it. Leptin was an important first step in unraveling the complex machinery by which the body regulates weight. It was also an object lesson in the overconfidence of some medical researchers and in the public's naive willingness to believe them.

The leptin story was unusual because the drug's reputation was created—and destroyed—by careful scientific research. More commonly, both doctors and patients are influenced by a more primitive and inherently misleading kind of evidence—the personal testimonial. Whether drugs are beneficial, toxic, or completely ineffective, legions of doctors and patients emerge with testimonials about their value. Listen to the persuasive power of this true testimonial about Prozac, the best-selling drug for depression. It comes from a member of a support group for patients who have taken antidepressants.[13]

Glenn St. John of Vancouver, Canada, was prescribed Prozac for depression he suffered after his father died suddenly. "Prozac has been a godsend. I felt great—better than I felt in a long time," he said. "My work performance got better. My friends noticed as well." Even his mother saw positive changes. Under the influence of the drug, she observed, a long-standing negative streak had disappeared. He started sleeping better and began to lose some of his forty pounds of excess weight.

Psychiatrist Peter D. Kramer's best-selling book, *Listening to Prozac*, was built around similar dramatic stories. Prozac, he wrote, "seemed to give social confidence to the habitually timid, to make the sensitive brash, to lend the introvert the social skills of the salesman." Such gushing testimonials and media coverage helped make Prozac a best-seller, generating more than a billion dollars a year in sales for Eli Lilly.[14]

Kramer makes Prozac sound miraculous. What about the risks? Kramer's book is highly reassuring. "Prozac has few immediate side effects" (page 12). It "is a clean drug" (page 63). It is "a designer drug, sleek and high tech"[15] (page 64). The reader has to persevere all the way to page 206 to read about two patients who experienced side effects. Both were minor and resolved quickly.

When the manufacturer Eli Lilly claimed Prozac was mostly free of side effects, the FDA immediately objected. Such claims were "inconsistent with the product labeling that states 15% of the patients in clinical trials discontinued due to adverse experiences," the FDA said.[16] The FDA demanded that Lilly stop making such unfair claims. In fact, the label disclosure statement shows that Prozac has been linked to an astounding 242 different side effect, including 34 different medical problems in the genital and urinary tract alone. Over a ten-year period Prozac was associated with more hospitalizations, deaths, or other serious adverse reactions reported to the FDA than any other drug in America.[17] Two similar drugs for depression, Paxil and Zoloft, are of similar toxicity.[18]

Those who "listen to Prozac" and similar drugs more closely will hear stories such as these: "I felt a gentle lift soon after taking the first one," reported James Smith. "After a week, I started to feel mentally overheated, then jittery and increasingly anxious. By the following day, I just wanted to keep sleeping so I didn't have to face the trauma of being awake."

"I have been on Prozac about a year and am feeling a lot better," reported Kelly James. "The only real problem I have experienced is a complete lack of emotion."

"Has anyone had orgasm side effects with Paxil?" Sara Huzford asked members of a support group. "The depression is gone but also the orgasms. It's driving me and my husband crazy. I started on Prozac. No depression, but nausea and terrible shakes. Tried Zoloft, definitely no orgasm. Paxil limits me to one a month if I am lucky. Do I need to choose between my sex life or depression?"

Something is seriously wrong with a system in which both doctors and patients embrace antidepressants so uncritically when the scientific record shows they have few equals in their capacity to produce unpleasant and sometimes dangerous adverse effects.

Books, scientific studies, and media reports about the dangers of drugs trigger a hostile and vigorous defense from doctors and drug companies. Through bitter experience, they have learned that if the bubble of rosy expectations bursts, consumer trust can evaporate almost overnight. It is almost as if public attitudes toward prescription drugs are regulated by an oddly engineered pendulum that is never in proper balance. It leaps only from the extreme of unrealistic hopes to the opposite, a mindless terror about drugs. However, the commonsense strategy of trying to avoid "dangerous" drugs and only take the "safe" drugs is not a workable approach.

One of the most deadly poisons routinely available to the public can be found in any large supermarket among household goods. It is closely related to a chemical called warfarin, and used as rat poison.[19] However, warfarin is a lifesaving drug. It is available in prescription form as DuPont's Coumadin. Each year it is used 3 million times in office medical practice—more frequently than Valium or Tagamet.[20] In high-risk patients, it can prevent strokes by stopping dangerous blood clots from forming in the heart and in the legs.

Given the same chemical, what is the difference between rat poison and a lifesaving drug? Only the systematic testing in clinical trials that proved that for one carefully defined medical purpose, the benefits of rat poison clearly outweigh its risks. That lengthy and expensive testing doesn't make Coumadin "safe" so that people can take it freely. It can cause gangrene, fatal internal hemorrhaging, hideous birth defect, and life-threatening allergic reactions. Its anticlotting effects must be carefully monitored with laboratory tests.[21] Nevertheless, for specifically defined medical conditions, Coumadin has benefits that greatly outweigh its risks. Numerous other deadly poisons have important medical uses. Botulism toxin can relieve certain painful, body-contorting muscle spasms.[22] A chemical relative of curare is used to immobilize skeletal muscles for heart surgery.[23] Potassium chloride, lethal in large doses, can be essential to restore the chemical balance in patients taking drugs to eliminate excess body fluids.[24]

There is no such thing as a safe drug. However, hundreds of powerful drugs have great value for carefully defined medical uses in which benefits have been proven to greatly outweigh risks. The wise use of prescription drugs begins with this basic idea. Since the ancient Greeks, humans have dreamed of medicines so powerful they could make illness vanish. This was how a daughter of the Greek god of medicine came to be named Panacea. Thirty centuries later, the public still yearns for a panacea. Unfortunately, as the widespread use of Ritalin in children shows, drugs are frequently given as if they were a panacea rather than what they are—a tricky balance of risks and benefits.

Ritalin is a powerful brain stimulant with effects similar to cocaine and the amphetamines.[25] However, in children it has a calming effect. Given Ritalin, children sit more calmly and quietly in class.[26] They have less spontaneity in speech and thought, but focus better on assigned tasks. On short-term measures of attention and retention, they do better.[27] Ritalin or the amphetamines work on all kinds of children, not just those officially labeled with a medical disorder. The effects of Ritalin can be observed in normal children selected for superior academic performance and good relationships with peers.[28] They can also be seen in the mentally retarded.[29] So it is no surprise that similar effects can also be observed in children classified as hyperactive, or, in modern medical jargon, with attention deficit hyperactivity disorder.[30] The ability of Ritalin to suppress rowdy behavior in children is much more consistent than, for example, the effects of Prozac among the depressed. Uncounted thousands of grateful parents can attest to this quieting effect—a behavioral change well documented in systematic study.

Enthusiasts for drug treatment often claim hyperactivity in children is a "biochemical imbalance," apparently corrected by Ritalin. While such speculation may be plausible, researchers cannot identify which chemicals are involved, or find abnormal levels in the afflicted children. The chemical imbalance theory has not been established by scientific evidence.[31] The manufacturer declares, "The mode of action in man is not completely understood. Ritalin presumably activates the brain stem arousal system and cortex."[32] Translated into plain English, the manufacturer appears to have concluded that Ritalin "presumably" affects the brain. A drug whose chemical effects are uncertain is being given to children with a condition that cannot be precisely defined and is of unknown cause.

When careless thinking about benefits is combined with scientific ignorance about long-term effects, society can end up taking truly appalling risks. Ritalin is being given to almost 10 percent of school-age boys for short-term control of behavior—not to reduce any identifiable hazard to their health.[33] Such large-scale chemical control of human behavior has not been previously undertaken in our society outside of nursing homes and mental institutions.[34] What kind of risks may be involved?

The first concern about Ritalin is serious or irreversible side effects. The best documented problem is a form of brain damage called Tourette's syndrome. It causes tics, twitching, and abnormal sounds or movement, sometimes of a bizarre nature. The manufacturer, Novartis, says it has received "rare reports" of Tourette's syndrome among children taking Ritalin.[35] One research group kept score on 122 consecutive cases of children prescribed Ritalin, finding one child in which the brain damage was permanent.[36] However, 12 children had less severe tics or other abnormal movements for at least short periods of time. In the case where Tourette's syndrome persisted even after the child stopped taking the drug, the child's face twitched, his head turned back and forth abnormally, he smacked his lips incessantly, wiped his forehead, and made guttural sounds. In the less severely affected children, however, the eye rolling, throat clearing, eye bugging and neck turning "usually" involved temporary episodes. Another researcher found indications of abnormal movements or compulsive behaviors in 76 percent of the boys studied, although the effects were characterized as "often subtle and transient."[37] More common side effects reported in another Ritalin study were loss of appetite in about 40 percent, insomnia in 20 percent, and stomachaches in 20 percent.[38] The appetite suppression effect of stimulants (amphetamines are still approved for weight loss in adults, but with dire warnings about addiction) naturally led to concerns that they might stunt a child's growth. The manufacturer acknowledges this possibility but declares "a causal relationship has not been established."[39] Even the seemingly reassuring studies give little comfort. One research group found an adverse effect during the first year of Ritalin use but not during the second year.[40] However, among 72 children in the study, only 14 had taken Ritalin for two full years without interruption, and their growth was compared to "expected values" estimated from a standard table.

Especially in developing children, a decision on Ritalin ought to be based on the long-term benefits and risks as much as its immediate effects. If Ritalin helped children arrive at high school with notably better skills in reading and math, some parents might willingly accept the limited risks of brain damage or stunted growth. Thus, it should be of great concern to learn that the manufacturer of Ritalin declares, "Sufficient data on the safety and efficacy of long-term use of Ritalin are not yet available."[41] The medical literature is no more helpful. One of the leading textbooks deplores the lack of good long-term studies of academic performance, noting, "Those that have examined the issue have generally found negative results."[42] There is virtually no data on long-term side effects. Notes the textbook, "The deleterious effects of using stimulant medications over several years with children have not yet been well-studied."[43] Long-term safety is not an idle, theoretical question. Long after Ritalin had been approved, the federal government completed a study in 1995 showing it could cause cancer in mice. The overuse of Ritalin as a behavioral panacea has predictably led to other problems. The Drug Enforcement Administration has publicized it growing concerns about the outright abuse of this now universally available drug to get high.[44] It is astonishing that an uncritical nation has so enthusiastically embraced a drug that can cause cancer in animals, addiction in adults, brain damage in children, and whose long-term safety has not been established. We would be fortunate indeed if Ritalin were a unique case of failure to study long-term effects of drugs intended to be taken over the long term. In fact, prescription drugs are seldom evaluated for long-term effects, and the public health consequences of this glaring failure are truly frightening.

My previous book was an anatomy of the nation's worst prescription drug disaster so far. Over just a few years' time, an estimated 50,000 heart patients died from taking drugs for irregular heartbeats—drugs such as Tambocor, Enkaid, Mexitil, quinidine, and Procan.[45] Over the short term, these drugs had performed well, effectively suppressing mild irregular heartbeats. The theory was that over the long term, these otherwise harmless premature heartbeats might trigger life-threatening rhythm disruptions, even cardiac arrest. On this plausible but untested theory, doctors prescribed these drugs for hundreds of thousands of heart patients. In this case, however, the National Institutes of Health, using public money, sponsored a clinical trial to document the presumed long-term benefits of these drugs for irregular heartbeats. Some doctors even condemned the NIH for wasting money testing a medical treatment already widely accepted as beneficial by the nation's heart experts. The clinical trial had been under way for barely a year when researchers called an emergency halt in April 1989. They were shocked to discover they were giving patients drugs with some of the most lethal effects ever documented in clinical medicine. Two of these drugs—Tambocor and Enkaid—caused cardiac arrest in about 6 percent of the heart attack survivors who took them for one year's time. The assumed long-term health benefits simply did not exist. In a pattern that will be seen repeatedly, both drug companies and medical specialists vastly underestimated the risks of these drugs. They proved skillful in limiting the public outcry over this preventable medical catastrophe, and failed to come to terms with the size and consequences of this monumental medical error.

A hauntingly similar crisis began in the spring of 1995. This time the drugs at issue were the most widely used medicine in the entire world—a family of drugs called calcium channel blockers. They are prescribed for high blood pressure, and for the chest pains caused by heart disease. Two of the best-selling drugs in the United States are calcium channel blockers— Procardia XL (no. 8), and Cardizem CD (no. 11).[46] Others include Adalat, DynaCirc, Calan, Norvasc, Plendil, and Covera-HS. As usual, these drugs were tested and approved on the basis of short-term effects. They reduced blood pressure—a change most patients themselves could not detect or immediately benefit from. The hope was that over years of treatment these drugs would reduce the risk of stroke, and possibly of heart attack and death. In 1995, a string of disturbing medical studies began to appear. They showed that calcium channel blockers might increase the risk of heart attack or cancer—especially when compared to older, better-proven blood pressure drugs. Was it possible that 7 million Americans were taking a drug that was harming rather than improving their health? All this because no long-term testing was ever required? It was a failure of will, not a shortage of time or money. These drugs had $7 billion in worldwide sales and had been in clinical use for more than a decade. A tiny fraction of the profits would have paid for the necessary drug testing.

The evidence challenging the long-term safety of calcium channel blockers was extensive, credible, and deeply troubling, but not definitive.[47] In study after study, unexplained, excess deaths and other medical problems occurred among those taking various calcium channel blockers. One study found a greater risk of heart attack.[48] In another the problem was internal bleeding.[49] In two more studies, calcium channel blockers seemed to pose a higher risk of cancer.[50] Defenders of calcium channel blockers responded with a torrent of objections, mostly technical.[51] In this bewildering crossfire, very few focused on the central and uncontested fact. Here were the most widely prescribed drugs in the world, and no one had clear scientific evidence they were safe and effective for their intended long-term medical use. How sound is the system that fails to address so basic a question? Because of the enormous number of people taking calcium channel blockers, even a statistically small increase in risk could mean thousands of patient deaths.

Because so many millions are exposed, drugs have a potential for disaster that dwarfs most other risks of modern society. In the worst case, an automobile accident may claim several dozen lives. With a defective automobile design, hundreds may die. When a commercial airliner crashes, several hundred lives can be lost in the blink of an eye. With a defective aircraft design, the total could reach into the thousands. But in a prescription drug disaster, tens of thousands of people may die and literally millions are placed at risk. If calcium channel blockers injure only one-half of 1 percent of the people who take them each year, that still amounts to 35,000 casualties. Taking prescription drugs ranks as one of the most hazardous activities of modern society even though a majority of people who take them will not be harmed.

The typical response of the medical authorities to credible questions about drug safety is to reassure the patients, no matter what the actual dangers. The response to the first wave of public concern over calcium channel blockers was typical. The American College of Cardiology and the American Medical Association declared patients should "Assume these drugs are not dangerous to them."[52] Because of inadequate long-term drug testing, there was no evidence to support this assumption. The American Heart Association wanted patients now understandably worried about safety to do nothing. "They should not stop taking their medication but should consult their doctors," the group said. The drug companies, predictably, denounced the safety concerns as unfounded. They tried to calm doctors' concerns by stepping up marketing efforts and advertising. "Trust the experience," Pfizer said about best-selling Procardia XL.[53] Hoechst Marion Roussel declared it "stands firmly behind the safety and efficacy of the Cardizem family of products," and handed out packets of reassuring patient brochures for use in doctors' offices. If patients did call their doctors, they would encounter an industry-engineered message of reassurance. One frustrated defender of calcium channel blockers tried to halt the flow of studies about the dangers of these drugs by reminding doctors of the important but rarely spoken medical dictum, "Never Frighten Your Patients."[54]

Another example of reassuring the public at any cost still gives me nightmares. In the spring of 1983, alarm was spreading throughout the community of people with the blood-clotting disorder of hemophilia. Evidence was emerging that the then newly discovered HIV virus was apparently transmitted through blood. Hemophiliacs take clotting factor drugs made from human blood. Drug companies were quietly withdrawing the first batches of clotting drugs suspected of contamination with HIV. Amid this first flurry of public and professional concern, the National Hemophilia Foundation issued this urgent advisory to the chapters serving the national's 14,000 affected persons: "Public media coverage of AIDS is causing some patients to abandon appropriate use of blood products because they fear contracting AIDS. The NHF AIDS task force considers this to be an inappropriate response and urges hemophiliacs to maintain use of clotting factor in their treatment of hemorrhagic episodes."[55] By the end of 1984, at least half of the nation's hemophiliacs were infected with HIV. Thousands have already died and many more will succumb. No one knows how many of those lives might have been saved if the foundation had not yielded to the conventional policy of reassurance at any cost.

These are the troubling warning signs of a system that urgently needs major reform. How safe is a system that can't even count the deaths and serious injuries, let alone operate effective programs to prevent them? How sane is a system that provides mind-altering drugs to millions for decades without first establishing the long-term safety and benefits? How can we objectively weigh the risks and benefits of drugs when doctors and patients alike embrace new drug fads with an astonishing lack of healthy skepticism and critical thinking? Why do the health authorities almost invariably reassure patients—regardless of the actual risks—rather than taking effective measures to reduce those dangers? The coming chapters will explore the nature of powerful prescription drugs and explain why they must inevitably have substantial risks. Next, the book will examine the deeply flawed system created to manage and control these risks. Finally, it will examine what, as individuals and as a society, we can do to minimize these dangers. It will show that it is perfectly possible to embrace the great benefits of powerful prescription drugs without being so reckless about their substantial risks.

This book will likely be assailed by defensive doctors and angry drug companies. It is worth addressing in advance the predictable charges that have been used for many years to attack others who have dared to speak out about drug safety. Apologists often claim: "Sure, all drugs have side effects. This is just the price we must pay for the tremendous benefits of drugs." The fatal flaw in this argument is readily exposed by applying it to any other of society's major risks. Would anyone dare argue that a few dozen airplane crashes are the price we have to pay for the tremendous benefits of commercial air travel? Of course not. The public demands and gets action to insure that the risks of air travel are kept to an absolute minimum. The pages of this book will be packed with specific examples of unnecessary deaths and preventable injuries.

The claim that a million serious injuries is just the price we have to pay also implies the threat that if we ask too many questions about the safety of drugs, perhaps valuable medication will never be brought to market or will be restricted in some fashion. In fact, this book aims to increase information and choices open to consumers, not reduce them. However, society is correct to prohibit the marketing and sale of drugs until they have been tested thoroughly enough to establish their risks and benefits. If drugs have no benefits, then it is irresponsible to expose the public to them since they will only cause harm.

Critics are also likely to charge that this book may frighten a few people so badly they will refuse to take drugs that will truly benefit them. Others who have warned of drug dangers have been accused of hastening the deaths of patients who suffered a heart attack or some other event after stopping a prescribed medication.[56] It is true that many people tend to have not one but two unhealthy attitudes toward drugs: mindless fear and blind faith. This book cannot be expected to change human nature on either account.

Finally, it will likely be alleged that this book, in its relentless focus on the dangers of drugs, lacks balance, that it is somehow unfair. The purpose of this book should be clear from the outset. It examines the risks and the dangers of drugs, and how they may be reduced. It does not pretend to catalog or present all their health benefits. The drug industry spends more than $10 billion a year to promote drugs to doctors and consumers alike. An army of drug salesmen daily plies doctors with free samples, gifts, and snappy brochures touting drug benefits. Newspapers and the television news are filled with direct-to-consumer advertising. One of the major reasons why drugs are so unnecessarily hazardous today is that so much attention has focused on the benefits of drugs and so little has been devoted to understanding and reducing their risks.

CHAPTER TWO

Drug Safety

HOW SAFE ARE THE DRUGS you take? Many people are comfortable with the idea of dangerous drugs until they find one in their own medicine cabinet. Also, some consumers happily take drugs daily without expectations of great benefit. They hope the drugs will help them, but they rarely become disappointed or feel cheated if nothing much happens. It's hard to imagine a consumer upset with Merck because he had a heart attack despite taking Zocor for high cholesterol. (In fact, the manufacturer's data show two out of three heart attacks still will occur despite the drug.)[1] What many consumers do expect is that the drug won't hurt them, that they can be used reasonably freely without fear of injury. So how safe are the most frequently prescribed drugs taken every day by a majority of the adult population? "Safe" simply means free of danger or the risk of injury. Among the most commonly prescribed medications, how many safe drugs can be found? Do the drugs you take make the list?

This search for safe drugs will focus on the 50 most

frequently prescribed medications. In one year, they account for 28 percent of all prescriptions written, a total of more than 650 million bottles of medication, or almost three for every man, woman, and child in the United States.[2] These are the drugs for the most common medical disorders. Among the 50 best-sellers are 9 antibiotics, 8 drugs for high blood pressure, 6 drugs for pain, 5 hormones, and 5 drugs for depression or anxiety. The list also includes important drugs for ulcers, epilepsy, diabetes, heart disease, and prostate problems. The top-selling drugs are targeted against the most common medical disorders of modern humans. This means the market is large. Also, best-seller status means a drug has been successful in a highly competitive marketplace, winning acceptance by the FDA, physicians, and patients. In searching for a group of safe drugs, the top 50 are a logical place to start. While a few of the drugs—notably antibiotics and some painkillers—are used for a short course of treatment, the large majority are intended to be taken for months, if not years on end. Whatever their risks, tens of millions of people will be exposed to the most frequently prescribed drugs. In exploring the safety of these highly successful drugs, the central questions is: Can they be taken free of concern that they might cause death or a serious injury, or precipitate a potentially life-threatening medical crisis?

The first safety standard for the top 50 involves one of the oldest-known risks of drugs. Is taking them habit-forming, and can it lead to addiction or abuse? A truly safe drug would not be addictive—and a large majority of drugs are free of such a risk. However, the U.S. Drug Enforcement Administration has flagged 7 of the top 50 drugs for the addiction and abuse danger. They are subject to special government controls. They include painkiller drugs containing Darvon or propoxyphene, codeine and other opium derivatives such a hydrocodone. The DEA drug list also includes the anxiety medication Xanax (or its chemical equivalent, alprazolam). Each time you take a drug, it would be safer not to have to worry about taking a small step toward an addiction that might require lengthy and unpleasant treatment to overcome.

Cancer is the second safety concern for widely used drugs. Because drug therapy involves the body absorbing relatively large amounts of a powerful chemical, we would like assurances that these drugs do not cause cancer. There might be trace amounts of a suspected carcinogen in the pesticide residue on an apple, possibly a little more in the burnt material on a barbecued beefsteak. That exposure is tiny compared to swallowing several pills a day for months or years on end. Identifying any kind of chemical that might cause cancer is far from an exact science, but previous research suggests three kinds of widely accepted cancer warning flags.[3] We may be concerned if a drug:

- Causes cancer in humans.
- Causes cancer in animal testing.
- Damages the genetic material, causing cell mutations.

Animal studies and cell mutation assays are part of the standard testing of new drugs. It is, of course, unthinkable to do cancer testing in humans, but enough evidence has emerged to convince the experts about a few dozen chemicals. Among the top 50 drugs, human evidence of cancer risk is reported for 4 drugs, animal evidence implicates another 12 drugs, and an additional 2 caused cell mutations. Among the best-selling drugs, 19 were apparently not tested for cancer risk.[4] But let's give them the benefit of the doubt, counting only those drugs with scientific evidence of cancer risk. Therefore, 18 of the top 50 drugs have measurable cancer risks. Among the popular drugs with one of the above-noted cancer risks are Premarin, Mevacor, Dilantin, and Prilosec. These drugs provide benefits that may convince consumers to accept these cancer risks (if they even know about the danger). However, we can't call them safe drugs in the sense of being free of the risk of injury. When we remove from the list of safe drugs those with either addition potential or positive evidence of cancer risk, just 24 of the original top 50 are left.

Next, we might want to avoid drugs that are unusually toxic. Let's call "unusually toxic" any drugs that has been linked to more than 50 different side effects.[5] To meet the "unusually toxic" test, these many adverse effects must also occur so frequently that at least 10 percent of the patients discontinued the drug during testing. This standard immediately claims the three most popular antidepressants—Prozac, Zoloft, and Paxil. Each causes more than two hundred different adverse effects and is discontinued by about 15 percent of patients. A drug also qualifies as unusually toxic if it can create a potentially life-threatening medical emergency with little or no warning. This test claims all antibiotics that are based on penicillin. Approximately 5 percent of the population has an allergic reaction to penicillin, requiring lifelong vigilance by the individual—and the medical system. An allergic reaction can be unpleasant in many cases, and in very rare cases, lethal.[6] Without question, penicillin is one of the most valuable treatments in all of medicine. But penicillin can't be said to be safe, in the sense that it can be used freely and without concern for the risks—even though some people use it that way. The other potentially life-threatening emergency comes from two asthma drugs on the list—Proventil and Ventolin. Instead of relieving the symptoms of an asthma attack, these drugs are sometimes capable of unexpectedly producing a life-threatening bronchial spasm. The third and last test for unusual toxicity is dose. If a small overdose can lead to a medical emergency or life-threatening crisis, that is an important safety concern. An overdose could occur because a consumer forgets and takes an extra pill, or because some other factor or illness reduced the body's capacity to process or eliminate the drug. Among those drugs where a small overdose can cause serious medical problems are the popular antihistamine Seldane; the most widely used heart drug, Lanoxin, and Coumadin, the drug that prevents blood clots.[7] With all the unusual toxic drugs removed from the shrinking list, our search for a safe drug has now narrowed to just 14.

Finally, safe drugs ought to be free of adverse effects on the heart. Especially among the older population with many drug prescriptions, it could be dangerous to take a drug that causes a rapid heartbeat, a cardiac arrest, which can block the electrical signal to the heart to contract, or that contributes to other heart disorders. This standard eliminates all but 4 of the 14 remaining drugs. In fact, cardiac adverse effects are so widespread that this test would have eliminated 25 of the drugs all by itself.

While not any absolute guarantee of safety, it is interesting to examine the four survivors. Two are replacements for human hormones: insulin for diabetes, and Synthroid for those with medical problems caused by low levels of thyroid hormone. Also on the list is K-Dur, a potassium supplement given to people whose natural potassium levels are dangerously depleted by diuretic drugs. The final entry is Relafen, a painkiller and nonsteroidal anti-inflammatory drug. However, Relafen is part of a class of drugs whose hazards are important enough to warrant an entire chapter of this book.[8]

If we simply tally up the risks of the top 50, we discover that 7 cause addiction, 18 have cancer risks, 18 are unusually toxic, and 25 have cardiac risks.

These four basic safety tests—addiction, cancer risks, unusual toxicity, and cardiac effects—were arbitrarily selected because such information is reported for almost every drug. Also, these standards make intuitive good sense. However, it is not even close to a complete catalog of drug hazards. It is a more elaborate proof of the statement in the opening chapter: There is no such thing as a safe prescription drug. To hope for a safe drug is not a useful way to think about the problem. To avoid drugs altogether because of fear is to abandon their great benefits—which are occasionally lifesaving and frequently enhance the quality of life. Understanding that we can't have the drugs without the danger is the first step toward using them wisely and controlling their risks.

Some of those intimidated by the invasive power of modern drugs make the mistake of turning to natural remedies. The apparent logic is that chemicals found in the human body or in nature have to be gentler and healthier than the artificial products of modern chemistry. Not necessarily. Consider the natural human hormones. Estrogen, and a number of close chemical relatives, are proven carcinogens in humans.[9] A thyroid hormone (chemically different from the best-selling replacement hormone, Synthroid)[10] appeared to cause heart attacks in high-risk men, causing a major clinical experiment to be halted on safety grounds.[11] Through a loophole in the law created in 1994 by a Congress bent on curbing the FDA, some hormones are not subject to the same FDA regulation and exhaustive clinical testing as prescription drugs. However, rather than being more natural and gentler, human hormones are powerful chemical agents, having profound effects on the body's control system. Nevertheless, people have flocked to the inadequately tested hormones melatonin and DHEA.[12] Is it a mystery why people would agree to take two powerful hormones whose functions in the human body are not fully understood, when the therapeutic dose is unknown, and long-term safety and efficacy undocumented. These may have been the same people who wanted to take leptin, the new obesity hormone, before it had been tested in a single human being. Herbal remedies are more likely to be harmless than poisonous. However, notable exceptions have occurred. A manufacturing error in the amino acid L-tryptophan—taken to promote sleep—caused serious blood disorders.[13] Beta-carotene supplements have caused increased risk of cancer.[14] High doses of selenium or vitamin E may lead to serious health problems.[15]

With the top 50 prescription drugs, consumers get chemicals subject to FDA-mandated rigorous testing, established purity, scientifically documented benefits, and reasonably well-known risks at least over the short term. The top 50 are the most popular drugs, the fruits of the most advanced medical scientists, and, compared to herbal remedies, thoroughly tested. Then why do they remain so dangerous? Why hasn't a free market, billions of dollars, and a flourishing science produced drugs without these troubling risks? Why can't we have drugs that meet the basic human dream of something we can take freely without worrying about it? It turns out that the problems of prescription drugs are embedded in the very nature of how we think about and invent new medicines. The biology of how modern drugs work helps explains why modern drugs must be inherently unpredictable.

Imagine a single human cell so big that the outer membrane would stretch from the floor to the ceiling of a whole room. The flexible cell membrane is a busy place. Certain molecules—now the size of baseballs in our gigantic model—slip readily through the membrane into the cell. But molecules with other shapes bounce harmlessly off the slippery membrane and pass on their way. This particular human cell happens to be a factory making a chemical essential to the body. If we look closely, we will see a small pouch filled with the chemical move from inside the cell out through the membrane.

This cell became a chemical factory according to the genetic code of the DNA inside. But the cell still needs instructions about how much chemical to make, and when to release it. Embedded in the cell membrane are the control switches for this chemical factory. They are called cellular receptors. Each receptor switch can be triggered only by a specific chemical messenger, a molecule dispatched for this exact purpose. The classroom analogy is a lock and key, or perhaps an auto ignition switch and key. This particular cell has one receptor switch to increase output. If triggered, another may temporarily shut down the factory. In the cell wall are many other mysterious structures that seem to be other controls, but no one has yet figured out what they really do.

The basic idea of most modern drugs is disarmingly simple. They seek to control cell receptor switches. Some drugs turn the control switches to the ON position. They are call agonists. Other drugs interfere with the body's own chemical messengers. They occupy or block the cell receptor switch so the body can't change its setting. They are called blockers or antagonists. The antiulcer drug Tagamet is a blocker. In the cells lining the stomach are receptor switches. The body sends chemical messengers to turn the switches to the ON position, signaling the cells to secrete hydrochloric acid to help digest food. In some people, under some circumstances, the powerful acid can also damage or even perforate the stomach lining. Tagamet blocks the cell receptors so the cells don't receive the message to secrete acid.

There would be few dangerous drugs if the human body were a simple, tidy, rational engineering design. Then chemists could devise a molecule designed to match only the control switches for sleep, or anxiety, or sugar level. Unfortunately nature had other ideas. Consider the operation of one of the most familiar and best-researched chemical messengers—adrenaline, or in formal terms, epinephrine. We have all felt the adrenaline rush. It sounds the alarm and prepares the body to fight or flee. It is the work of a single chemical messenger, secreted by the small adrenal glands that sit on top of the kidney. But this single adrenaline messenger, throwing cell receptor switches all over the body, achieves a remarkable variety of effects. It makes the blood vessels near the skin constrict. (Why people turn white with fear.) But it makes blood vessels supplying the brain and the bronchial passages expand. Digestion is slowed, but the heart beats faster. Adrenaline, in fact, was isolated early in this century and its effects were so diverse that it had few medical uses.

In 1948, a key discovery about adrenaline laid the foundation for a breakthrough. A Georgia pharmacologist named Raymond Ahlquist learned that the body had two different kinds of receptor switches that responded to adrenaline.[16] He called them alpha- and beta-receptors. In general, alpha-receptors stimulated cells and speeded things up. Beta receptors tended to slow things down. Even so, this was not a consistent effect. The human heart, for example, was loaded with beta-receptors that normally inhibit cell actions. But in the heart, beta-receptors stimulated a faster heartbeat. Later researchers identified several different kinds of alpha- and beta-receptors. Probably no one has yet found them all. The same basic scheme seen in adrenaline works elsewhere. The body sends relatively few and simple commands through its chemical messengers. But the cells have an abundant variety of receptor switches to achieve all the millions of fine adjustments the body requires to respond to a constantly changing environment.

In 1962, a British physician and physiologist named James Whyte Black became the first person to understand that these cellular receptors could be exploited to make powerful medicines.[17] He focused on the medical problem called angina—the chest pains sometimes experienced by people with heart disease. The pains occur because the heart is temporarily starved for oxygen and nutrients. When the body calls for extra output from the heart, the network of tiny blood vessels that nourish the heart muscle are too clogged up to allow sufficient blood flow. From Ahlquist's work, Black also knew one precise mechanism by which the body commands the heart to beat harder and faster: Adrenaline stimulates the beta-receptors in the heart muscle. Black realized that if he could create a beta-blocker, it ought to prevent chest pains. With the receptors blocked, the heart would not respond to the chemical messenger adrenaline when it arrived with the command to beat harder and faster. The result was propranolol (sold in the United States as Inderal), a powerful heart drug that is widely used for angina, to prevent heart attacks, and to lower blood pressure. Typically, drugs do not block all the receptors entirely; at therapeutic doses they usually reduce the response rather than eliminate it.

The central idea—and the central problem of drugs—is cellular receptors. How is the colony of trillions of separate cells that we call a human body coordinated? Every thought, every fear, each chemical change, every twitch of an eyelash, and all memories are a product of cellular receptors. Receptors are what make complex organisms possible. Black's idea of controlling cell receptors with drugs was a discovery of profound importance. Chemists could now create drugs to send their own instructions to the cells or obstruct the body's own commands. This was the core idea of receptor-based drugs, of which Black's beta-blocker was the first of premeditated human design. However, like all new powers that humans have discovered, it opened the door to new dangers. These drugs were an unprecedented intervention into the delicately tuned, constantly changing chemical operations of the human body. It was chemical meddling in a system designed to exclude such interference. In harsher terms, it was turning lose a chemical bull in a human china shop.

Neither science nor real life is tidy, so notable drugs emerged that were not based on receptor theory. The mechanism of many valuable drugs remains unknown. General anesthesia is an example of such a mystery drug. Antibiotics are important and widely used, but they don't work through the receptors of human cells. By various strategies, they kill bacteria and other microbial predators. The cholesterol-lowering drug Questran never leaves the intestine. It removes cholesterol from the body by binding to the cholesterol-rich bile acid that circulates through the intestine to aid digestion. Exceptions aside, cell receptor theory was the controlling idea that drove an ever expanding pharmaceutical research establishment.

The profound implications of cell receptor drugs never captured the public imagination as did Einstein's theory of relativity or Watson and Crick's unraveling of the structure of DNA. While not everyone grasped the details of Einstein's theory, thoughtful people everywhere pondered a strange new world in which something as seemingly immutable as time turned out to be just another variable. For decades before anyone made practical use of DNA, people debated and feared the prospect of genetic engineering. But faithful to the ancient tradition of asking no questions about the prescribed drugs we take, we allowed these powerful agents based on control of cell receptors to spread into universal use with little understanding of the great revolution that had just occurred. With a minimum of public discussion, receptor theory drugs began to affect directly the lives of practically everyone. There were contraceptive pills, beta-blockers, calcium channel blockers; antihistamines like Hismanal and Claritin, and anti-inflammatory drugs like ibuprofen, Relafen, and Feldene. Receptor theory helped spawn—or explain—antidepressants such as Prozac and stimulants such as Ritalin. Even for useful drugs whose function remained a mystery, the research agenda often focused on identifying to which cellular receptors these drugs were bound, and how they worked.

Wonderful as this may be, cellular receptors also explain why modern drugs are inherently dangerous and unpredictable. Because control systems are not all that familiar to the majority of us who are not engineers, let's dig one layer deeper into the cell receptor idea with an analogy. We'll focus on one kind of control switch—a household thermostat. Instead of a drug molecule as messenger, we will use a primitive robot so stupid that all it can do is search tirelessly through the house looking for anything the exact size and shape of a thermostat. If the dumb robot finds a thermostat, it nudges the temperature setting upward. This is, in fact, how drugs work. Suppose the house becomes too cold. This seems like the perfect assignment for the robot, which circulates through the house looking for thermostats. Whenever it finds one, it will adjust the setting upward. Most of the time, this will warm up the house. However, it will also turn up the refrigerator, the hot-water heater, and the freezer. Usually, a small change in these other thermostats won't matter. However, in a few cases this might turn out to be harmful. Maybe the freezer was old and ailing, and all the frozen food melted after the thermostat was turned up. Or perhaps the hot-water heater was very efficient, and somebody got burned because the water was now too hot. If the furnace was old and already at maximum capacity, then the small thermostat change might push it over the brink and destroy it. If this dumb robot is the only tool available to change the thermostat settings, most people will still be happy to have it. The larger point, however, is that the whole approach is inherently limited. It is frequently going to produce undesirable effects; under some circumstances it can do substantial harm. Note that the robot is very simple and reliable—just like a drug molecule. It has a remarkably consistent effect. It will find every switch it can and make exactly the same change each time. But the control system it is interfering with is not at all simple, and the switch settings are being changed all the time. The drug is changing settings with blind robotic consistency in a system that is designed to operate with all kinds of sensors and feedback mechanisms to keep everything in tune. This is inherently dangerous. Many of the noxious medicines taken in ancient times probably never even got out of the digestive tract. Modern receptor-based drugs are potent; they get into blood circulation and start flipping control switches everywhere. Some of these multitude of changes produce effects that are unwanted or unexpected. They are called adverse effects.

To survey the adverse effects of drugs, let's start at the very top of the human body with hair on our head—and work our way methodically downward.[18] At least 287 approved drugs may cause the hair to fall out. Included are not only the expected anti-cancer drugs, but also birth control pills, drugs for high blood pressure and two antidepressants, Paxil and Elavil. Even Rogaine, a drug that makes some hair grow back in some balding people, can make the hair fall out in others. A total of 14 drugs are linked to deafness; 16 to blindness, and 42 may impair the sense of smell. Consider all the different effects drugs can have just on the human tongue. Elavil and 16 other drugs cause a black, hairy tongue. The antibiotic Geocillin may cause a furry tongue. A sore tongue can result from the cholesterol drug Questran and the migraine drug Imitrex. The sleep-aid Halcion is linked to a burning tongue. The heart drub Tambocor may cause a swollen tongue. Four other drugs cause "smoker's tongue." Perhaps the most unpleasant, most serious, and most common effect on the tongue is produced in many patients who take neuroleptic drugs for severe mental illness. Damage to the brain's ability to control muscles causes the tongue to protrude from the mouth, making speech difficult and the patient's appearance bizarre. For those whose tongue does not protrude, these same drugs can make the tongue wiggle uncontrollably in the mouth like a worm. This recitation could continue, organ by organ, until the mind is numb—through a catalog of more than 2,500 different side effects.

In addition to achieving unpredictable and sometimes undesirable effects, the whole cell receptor approach has another problem waiting to snare the careless thinker. Drugs such as the beta-blocker must be examined from two quite different viewpoints. The drug has a biological effect—blocking the beta-receptors. Black, however, was seeking a medical benefit—preventing chest pains—which was only vaguely related to the biological effect of blocking beta-receptors all over the body. With other receptor drugs, the medical health benefit is sometimes a miscellaneous by-product of a series of biological effects. For example, scopolamine is a drug that might prevent you from getting seasick.[19] That is the medical or health benefit. However, scopolamine blocks certain receptors throughout the entire parasympathetic nervous system—that is the biological effect. It happens that a few of those receptors are in the digestive tract, and if you take the drug, you may not get seasick. Other receptors are in the mouth, so a dry mouth is a typical unwanted biological effect. Similarly, amphetamines are powerful stimulants of the central nervous system. Appetite suppression—the desired medical effect—is just one by-product of a much broader biological intervention. As the years passed, even the knowledgeable researchers who developed such drugs began to confuse the biological effects of their receptor switch drugs with a genuine medical or health benefit for a sick person. As we shall see later, this confusion would have dire consequences to the health of tens of thousands of people. However, from the moment of creation, the cell receptor idea was trapped in a paradox from which it can never escape. A predictable and relatively certain biological effect—the throwing of cell receptor switches—will invariably have all kinds of unexpected medical consequences. Some of these will prove to be ugly surprises.

This chapter has sought to show that the adverse effects are inevitable, inherently unpredictable, amazingly varied, and caused by most drugs. However, it still leaves an important question unanswered: How often do adverse effects occur, particularly those that cause serious injury, disability, or death? That is the subject of the next chapter.

CHAPTER THREE

The Dangers of Drugs

ON A GOLDEN DAY in October 1988, Lexi and John Mudd could count plenty of reasons to celebrate their seventeen years of marriage. The list would begin with their three daughters—the quiet and intellectual Alyssa, age fourteen; Sasha, already confident and outgoing at twelve, and Emily, eight, lover of animals. They lived in a century-old farmhouse that stood in the shadow of towering sequoia trees on what once was the largest estate in northern California. John Mudd, forty-six, was a psychiatrist with a practice in San Francisco. Mudd had a passion for exercise, playing squash and tennis regularly, biking at every opportunity. He had an identical twin, Tom, who also lived near San Francisco and owned a winery.

For their anniversary, Lexi and John had treated themselves to a weekend alone in the gently rolling hills of the Sonoma Valley. On this perfect Saturday morning in October, the hillside meadows had turned to gold, and the vineyards were beginning to lose their leaves. It was not surprising that John Mudd's idea of a good time was to get some serious exercise.

They would join two other couples and bike together over the steep, winding ten-mile grade from the Napa Valley to the Sonoma Valley. That would be followed by a gala dinner at a favorite Italian restaurant.

Lexi Mudd, suffering from some flulike symptoms, decided not to make the bike trip. In fact, Lexi didn't want her husband to make the arduous journey either. For several years, John had been suffering from an annoying but minor heart problem. The human heart has two small primer pumps, called the atria, that sit atop the powerful ventricles. A fraction of a second before each main contraction begins, the two small atria contract, squirting extra blood into the almost full main pumping chambers. John Mudd suffered from brief episodes of a condition called atrial fibrillation. Rather than contracting in a smooth, coordinated pulse, the muscle fibers become electrically disorganized and twitch chaotically. Because the larger ventricles are electrically isolated from the smaller atria, this disorder has little effect on the main pumping chambers. Typical symptoms are a feeling of fatigue, or a fluttering sensation in the chest. In John's case, the atrial fibrillation would vanish as suddenly and mysteriously as it had appeared. Other men might have rested during episodes of atrial fibrillation. John Mudd didn't even take a break from his squash game. However, as these attacks became more annoying and more frequent, Mudd had seen a cardiologist in San Francisco. The doctor had prescribed the heart drug Tambocor. Mudd started taking Tambocor just ten days before his bike ride up the steep grade between the Napa and Sonoma Valleys.

Tambocor was a problem from the start. John just didn't seem to feel as well as usual. After he brushed his teeth, John would always do ten chin-ups on the bar he had mounted in the bathroom. After taking Tambocor, he couldn't seem to do them. John had gone back to the cardiologist for new tests, but results weren't yet available. For this reason, Lexi didn't want John to make the bike trip. John thought this caution was unnecessary. Although he was a doctor himself, he had gone to a specialist, who had expressed no such concerns. So the trip was on, and Lexi drove the group over to the Napa Valley to begin the bike ride.

Much of life seems to be spent in an unchanging and predictable rut. However, such periods of seeming stability are punctuated by moments when the entire course of a lifetime can be changed by the tiniest and most seemingly inconsequential events. On this day in October, five people started up the hill toward Sonoma, and two of them were doctors—John, and Mark Levy, a psychiatrist who had gone through advanced training with John. However, Levy had a flat tire just minutes after they started, and dropped out. The other four continued onward and upward, leaving the only other doctor behind.

Just fifteen minutes later, John Mudd stopped riding. He got off his bike. He said he didn't feel well. Then he lay down beside the road and lost consciousness. Within minutes, the other man in the group was giving him CPR. On a hillside in the Napa Valley, CPR alone wasn't going to save John Mudd, but it could pry open a tiny window of opportunity. Through that tiny window drove one, lone passing car. In an incredible stroke of good fortune, the car was driven by an emergency room doctor who had just finished a shift at a nearby hospital. He had his kit with him. John Mudd was getting advanced care within minutes of his collapse. Ten minutes later, an ambulance arrived.

By the time Lexi got back to the motel, a message was already waiting telling her to go immediately to the hospital. Their friends had even summoned a taxi, which was waiting at the motel. When she reached the hospital, John was already stabilized, a heart rhythm restored, and on a respirator in the intensive care unit. However, he had not yet regained consciousness. The medical response had been so fast and so effective that everybody could still hope. The whole family gathered at the hospital to watch and wait.

The hospital completed a battery of extensive tests the next day. John Mudd's cardiac function looked increasingly strong. But he remain unconscious. The tests showed severe anoxia—irreversible damage from the minutes the brain was deprived of oxygen. The gathered clan talked about what to do now. "The facts were clear," Lexi remembered. "But it was hard to hear this news and understand the implications of it." They decided to transfer John to a bigger hospital in Marin County near their home. Another set of tests were performed. The results were unchanged. John Mudd's heart still lived. But his conscious brain was dead. On the sixth day after the bicycle ride, the family had to make one of the most difficult decisions that life ever demands of anyone. They agreed that John Mudd should be disconnected from the life support equipment.

Before that happened, Lexi took each of her girls, one by one, into the hospital room to say goodbye to their father. Sasha brought a long letter she had written. Now realizing her father was never going to read this letter, she taped it to his hand. Emily and Alyssa brought pieces of their baby blankets to tie around his fingers. When all the farewells were said, the life support equipment was removed. For another twenty-four hours, John Mudd's heart continued to beat. Then, without feeling pain or ever regaining consciousness, he died.

His twin brother, Tom, will never forget it. "He was my best friend for forty-six years." he said. "We were crib mates. We were very close. I don't think I was damaged. However, unless you have actually sat down and watched a twelve-year-old crying her heart out, you don't know what it's like." Lexi's life was never again the same. She later sued the 3M Company, which manufactures Tambocor, and won a damage settlement. Following an industry policy that helps conceal the harm drugs do, 3M paid damages only on condition that the size of the settlement remain confidential.

The ability of Tambocor and either similar drugs to cause cardiac arrest raised so many questions in my own mind that I wrote a book about it.[1] In an appendix, I sought to measure the casualties. As noted earlier, I estimate that these drugs for irregular heartbeats killed approximately 50,000 heart patients over just a few years' time.[2] However, the likely death toll was of such mind-numbing size that it seemed the only people who truly believed the totals were a handful of medical specialists who had the training to do the horrible arithmetic for themselves but had personally played no role in the tragedy. It is a major hazard all by itself that so many people cannot comprehend the magnitude of the dangers of drugs. Many doctors don't even like to mention the many risks of drugs, fearing that patients won't take them or that worry about side effects will slow their recovery.[3] An auto accident that claimed the father of three young girls might have been on the front page in the local newspaper. If Mudd had been on an airplane that crashed, his story would have been national news. But the victims of prescription drugs—even numbered in thousands—are seldom noticed and rarely reported. They are abandoned as an unpleasant fact of life that too many people would rather not face. As this chapter will show, it is harder to understand why so few people are concerned than to calculate the likely number of people who are killed or seriously injured by prescription drugs.

In modern societies, prescription drugs pose one of the greatest human-created dangers outside of war. Drugs are a preeminent hazard whether measured by their potential to cause catastrophe or by counting the annual toll of casualties from hundreds of different drugs. Also, society does some very risky business—such as erecting the steel skeletons of skyscrapers—but these dangers are confined to a small group of trained specialists. We set much, much lower safety thresholds for risks to which nearly the whole population is exposed. This is the case with prescription drugs. When millions are exposed, victims could number in the thousands even for a hazard that is, in statistical terms, very small.

The task of ranking prescription drugs among society's ongoing risks begins with the most direct and simple approach. Just count the severe injuries and deaths. Whether we are worrying about the victims of domestic violence or wondering whether the Air Force needs a better air safety program, a hard count of the victims is a sensible place to start. However, what ought to be an elementary check of the safety data turns out to require careful detective work and, unfortunately, some leaps of inference, intuition, and faith.

A risk-averse society normally tracks most of life's important accident risks with care. As a result, government records show 66 workers died in railway accidents in 1992.[4] Another 626 people died from electrical current in 1991, and 3,291 were killed by falls of less than one story.[5] However, when it comes to deaths and serious injuries caused by prescription drugs, neither the FDA nor any other federal health agency collects such information; no public or responsible private organization publishes regular estimates based on a consistent estimating method. Within the research community, there exists no consensus and very little literature about how to create a reasonably accurate total. Therefore, it becomes necessary to assemble a coherent picture from the fragmentary information available.

In some patients, widely used drugs set off life-threatening allergic reactions, disrupt the heartbeat, destroy most of the white blood cells, trigger episodes of bizarre behavior, damage the liver, create painful gallstones, or induce massive internal bleeding.[6] Such severe adverse effects require immediate and substantial medical attention, typically hospitalization. As it happens, hospitals are among the most carefully studied of medical institutions. Among the thousands of hospital studies in the scientific literature, some focus on admissions for adverse drug reactions. To stand at the door of any hospital to count how many entering patients had a disorder caused by prescription drugs provides a snapshot of the ongoing casualty toll. Also, it is reasonable to describe as "severe" any injury so serious that it required hospitalization.

Creating such snapshots has proved to be an appealing research project for ambitious young physicians seeking to build a record in research as well as patient care. Starting from a stack of hospital records as large as the researchers could stand, a team could count how many hospital admissions were caused by adverse drug reactions, and how many were caused by illnesses of some other origin. In 1966, at the dawn of the era of powerful prescription drugs, a team at Johns Hopkins University in Baltimore calculated that of 900 patients admitted to the medical service in one year, 3.5 percent were caused by adverse drug reactions.[7] More than fifty of these snapshot studies are in the medical literature beginning in 1960 and extending to the present day. In Montreal, 6.6 percent of all admissions were drug-related[8]; in Gainesville, Florida, 5.5 percent.[9] In Nampa, Idaho, 7.4 percent were caused by drugs.[10] A few studies focused on specialized hospital units. Pediatric intensive care units in Detroit, Boston, and Tulsa had a combined rate of 0.2 percent—the lowest reported.[11] However, a survey of pediatric cancer patients in those same cities showed prescription drugs caused 21.7 percent of admissions—the highest reported.[12]

Estimating total serious injuries is like trying to calculate the crowd at a Fourth of July parade based on a stack of amateur photos of the floats and various family members. You can't be certain that the photos reflect the crowd all along the route; it's possible that in some places the crowds might be more thickly packed or unusually sparse. Also, the various investigators used different rules to decide what was a hospital admission caused by an adverse drug reaction. (However, almost all excluded illegal drugs and intentional overdoses.) Finally, the drugs in clinical use changed substantially from when the studies began in 1960 to the present day. But in all studies the medical condition caused by drugs was so severe it warranted hospital admission.

The most comprehensive overview comes from a medical journal report that combined the worldwide results of thirty-six such studies covering forty-nine hospitals—every suitable peer-reviewed study in the world scientific literature. The author, Thomas Einarson of the University of Toronto, concluded that drugs account for an average of 5.1 percent of hospital admissions.[13] I focused on eight of the best and most consistent studies in the United States and got the same result, 5.1 percent. A Vanderbilt University expert in biostatistics reviewed the literature and estimated prescription drugs caused 3 to 5 percent of hospital admissions.[14] In 1993, FDA Commissioner David A. Kessler, writing in *JAMA*, the journal of the American Medical Association, estimated adverse drug reactions accounted for 3 to 11 percent of hospital admissions.[15] The highest incidence estimate was seen in a study from the Center for Pharmaceutical Economics, which estimated 11 to 28 percent of hospital admissions might have been related to prescription drugs.[16]

Taking even the lowest estimate—3 percent—yields an appalling overall toll from prescription drugs. It means 1 million people severely injured every year.[17] The same data suggest about 60,000 deaths.[18] The Pharmaceutical Research and Manufacturers of America, PhRMA, recently estimated an even higher annual total—1.3 million hospitalizations per year and 63,000 deaths.[19] The industry figure appeared in a position paper on drug safety that assailed as exaggerated another estimate of up to 2 million annual hospitalizations. In truth, the scanty, fragmentary data are not complete enough to tell which estimate is correct. I selected a very conservative total to avoid a distracting debate on estimating techniques. All these counts also omit important categories of serious drug injuries and disabilities that typically don't result in hospitalization. For example, thousands of people suffer from drug-induced symptoms of Parkinson's disease, and hundreds of thousands of others experience disabling effects from drugs for severe mental illness. Also, the researchers could only count well-known, well-documented adverse effects of drugs. As we shall see later, serious and even lethal adverse effects of major drugs have gone undetected for decades. For this chapter, the estimate merely has to be accurate enough to rank the overall danger of prescription drugs among other major risks of modern society.

No other cause of accidents in our society even approaches an annual toll of a million severe injuries. The largest competing accident hazard is automobile accidents, which injure about 95,000 people every year severely enough to require hospitalization.[20] That means you are ten times more likely to be put in the hospital by prescription drugs than because of an automobile accident. Put another way, each person has a 26 percent lifetime risk that a prescription drug will cause an injury severe enough to require hospitalization.[21] Here is a table that ranks common lifetime risks:

NATURE OF HAZARD	LIFETIME RISK
Severely injured by prescription drugs	26 in 100
Smokers' risk of lung cancer death	9 in 100
Severely injured in auto accident	2 in 100

Murder	1 in 100
Killed in commercial air crash	1 in 35,000
Struck by lightning	1 in 70,000

These estimates do not include another major source of drug-induced injuries—those occurring in the nation's hospitals. Earlier, hospital admission was used as a measure of severity. Another group of important studies focus on adverse drug reactions among patients in the course of their regular hospital treatment—regardless of why they were admitted in the first place. In the hospital environment, multiple drugs are used in aggressive treatment—with a patient typically getting ten to fifteen drugs during a hospital stay.[22] The intravenous route for administering many of these drugs makes adverse effects occur more rapidly and with greater severity. The clearest and most chilling snapshot of drug risks during hospitalization comes from a study of two Harvard-affiliated hospitals, Massachusetts General and Brigham and Women's.[23] The investigators reported adverse drug episodes in 6.5 percent of the patients treated—a frightening total indeed. (Remember the 26 percent figure was a *lifetime* risk over seventy years' time; this 6.5 percent risk occurs over an average seven-day hospital stay.)[24] Of these adverse drug episodes, 1 percent were fatal and 12 percent were life-threatening. If we assume that all the nation's 6,200 hospitals are operated with quality control standards similar to these two famed Boston teaching hospitals, then each year about 2 million people are injured by drugs while hospitalized, and about 20,000 killed.[25] A Harvard team featuring many of the same researchers also studied the most severe adverse events occurring in New York State hospitals.[26] Extrapolating to the entire nation, their results suggest that in one year medical drug errors caused 200,000 people to be disabled for six months or more and resulted in more than 30,000 deaths.

Summing up the deaths estimated from these two kinds of studies—hospital admissions for drug reactions and those incidents occurring during hospital care, the death toll reaches approximately 100,000 persons per year. Recent studies in peer-reviewed journals also cite an estimate of 140,000 annual deaths.[27] Normally, death data are more reliable than estimates of injury because, unless drugs are responsible, accidental deaths are independently investigated. In this case, however, information about drug-related deaths is notably less reliable than the information about injuries. Most of the individual hospital studies had only a handful of deaths, sometimes just one. Calculating national event rates from such data is pushing estimation toward its limits. Even if we assume that drugs claim as few as 70,000, and possibly more than 140,000 lives, where do prescription drugs rank among other lethal hazards of life? This tally focuses on deaths from accidents and other human activity rather than natural causes and disease.

CAUSE OF DEATH	ANNUAL DEATHS[28]
All causes	2,286,000
Prescription drugs	100,000
Auto accidents	42,000
Suicide	31,000
Murder	26,000
On-the-job accidents	4,000
Commercial air travel	67*

*The index year 1993 was followed by a year with 328 deaths.

With 100,000 annual deaths, 1 million severely injured, and another 2 million harmed during hospitalization, adverse reactions to drugs rank as one of the greatest man-made dangers in modern society. All these estimates are likely to underestimate the harm that prescription drugs cause. The casualty toll rises dramatically as researchers look more thoroughly and effectively for evidence. For example, the official records of the United States—data from death certificates—show that in 1991 just 163 deaths resulted from "drugs, medicaments, and biological substances causing adverse effects in therapeutic use."[29] More than ten times as many adverse-effect deaths were voluntarily reported to the FDA—a total of 1,806 deaths.[30] Even this is only a small fraction of the realistic estimate of 100,000 deaths a year. Who knows what a careful, systematic study might reveal.

The totals above also understate the true extent of harm because they omit an entire category of drug injuries that surely must number in millions. There is simply not enough evidence in the scientific record to support a plausible estimate of those who are injured severely enough to see a doctor but do not require hospitalization. What all this evidence does prove is that so many people are routinely injured by prescription drugs in our society today that it constitutes a major uncontrolled peril. The more rigorously the risk of prescription drugs is examined, the higher the resulting total of deaths and serious injury.

One of the most important dangers of prescription drugs may not be reflected in any single year's accident totals. A researcher checking admissions to a hospital might not see a single case. The only hint might be an uncertain warning in a medical journal about the unusual adverse effects of some new drug. Nevertheless, without warning, the most serious of modern industrial accidents may still be occurring—a medical catastrophe in which thousands are severely injured by the unexpected adverse effect of a single drug.

Prescription drugs make the very short list of threats that can injure a thousand or more people in a single episode. A plague can do it, as can a war or nuclear reactor meltdown. An aircraft design defect that caused several crashes could kill a thousand people. A chemical plant or toxic gas might get out of control. But these are the kinds of threats against which society erects its most effective defenses, and, in general, catastrophic accidents are rare in advanced industrial democracies. One troubling exception is prescription drugs and therapeutic products from human blood products. Catastrophic accidents occur repeatedly with prescription drugs, and society's defenses seem never quite good enough. A look at the unique features of major drug disasters reveals why.

There are few catastrophic risks in modern society to which so many people are exposed. An industrial fire, a refinery explosion, an aircraft prone to crash under certain conditions, can result in catastrophe. But relatively few people are exposed to these risks. But hundreds of thousands of people are routinely exposed to a moderately successful drug, and millions might take a blockbuster. Once such example is the catastrophe involving DES (diethylstilbestrol), the synthetic sex hormone given to 4.8 million pregnant women in what turned out to be the mistaken belief that it might help prevent spontaneous abortions, miscarriage, or premature birth.[31] Many of the children of mothers given DES developed abnormal growths on their sexual organs, cancer, and infertility. Because of the widespread use over decades, the victims are numbered in the hundreds of thousands. Even drugs that harm fewer than 1 in 100 can still produce tens of thousands of preventable injuries.

In a drug catastrophe, it is often an important challenge simply to find the victims. For more than a decade a drug called phenformin was given to hundreds of thousands of people with mild elevations of blood sugar, a condition called Type 2 or noninsulin-dependent diabetes. Phenformin reliably lowered blood sugar levels toward the normal range. For years, doctors were puzzled by cases of a strange disorder called lactic acidosis. When blood circulation is inadequate through muscle fibers, lactic acid concentrations increase. Lactic acidosis can also occur in heat stroke when exercise is involved. The drug phenformin was causing dangerous buildups of lactic acid. In someone who is ill, there are usually many suspects, and phenformin was only one of them. Thousands of patients died before phenformin was banned as an imminent danger to health in 1977. Had even a small fraction of the phenformin victims been killed in a single crash, storm, or explosion, the problem would have been spotted instantly, the cause quickly determined. But drug catastrophes tend to be slow, insidious, and difficult to see.

Prescription drugs also operate on the dangerous boundary between knowledge and ignorance. It is from ventures into the unknown that promising advances are produced, and from that same territory that new catastrophic threats also emerge. Even when the effects of the drug are simple and readily characterized, the human organism in which they work remains poorly understood. This was clearly illustrated in the catastrophe involving a moderately rare disorder of infants. Every year, thousands of newborns develop an allergy to milk, wheat, and corn. The solution is a special soybean-based infant formula. In the late 1970s, the main product for this market was called Neo-Mullsoy. After months of giving their babies Neo-Mullsoy, mothers around the country began noticing that their babies were different. They were developing more slowly, not talking or walking when expected. In the early stages, it wasn't even clear that anything was wrong. But in fact, a catastrophe was occurring. Responding to a health fad of the period, Neo-Mullsoy was sold as a "salt free" product during a time in which many experts were telling the public that table salt was dangerous. It was a tragic mistake. We now know that brains of babies do not develop normally without the chloride found in salt. As a result, thousands of babies will never reach their full potential. While technically Neo-Mullsoy was not a drug, it was a product sold by Syntex, a drug company, for a specific medical condition, and with the same catastrophic risks as prescription drugs. Even though salt is one of the most elementary of chemicals, a developing baby's brain is a complex mechanism that science does not fully understand.

In the most troubling of the drug catastrophes, unexpected evidence emerges that thousands of people are being injured, but the drugs remain in use because no satisfactory replacements exist. The classic example is the family of drugs called neuroleptics—given to people suffering from schizophrenia, and other severe disorders that involve visions, paranoia, delusions, mysterious voices urging bizarre acts, and other extremes of abnormal behavior. Neuroleptic drugs have been widely hailed for their capacity to permit many of the mentally ill to return to the community. What the public has been much slower to understand is that these same drugs also constitute a kind of toxic chamber of horrors. "Neuroleptic"—the medical term for these drugs—means "capable of damaging the nervous system." A majority of patients experience side effects. These include a condition called dystonia, in which some muscles contract painfully, forcing the body into tortured positions. "Acute dystonic reactions are terrifying to patients; sudden death has occurred in some instances," notes a leading pharmacology textbook.[32] Even more alarming is a condition called akathisia, an extreme form of agitation in which patients feel the need to move constantly and endlessly. In extreme cases, akathisia can be so painful that patients commit suicide to escape it.[33] Worse yet, psychiatrists often mistake the agitated behavior for a sign of mental illness and increase the dose.[34] But the most common adverse effects are called tardive dyskinesia and reflect damage to an area of the brain that controls voluntary muscle movements. Notes a major text, "Tardive dyskinesia is characterized by stereotyped, repetitive, painless, involuntary, tic-like movements of the face, eyelids, mouth, tongue, extremities or trunk."[35] Put simply, this is brain damage, and with longer-term exposure to these drugs, it becomes irreversible. It is the most widespread adverse effect of neuroleptic drugs, with estimates as low as 15 percent and as high as 70 percent in some populations.[36] With 3 million to 5 million people taking neuroleptic drugs, and therapy typically continuing over many years, these drugs must have caused far more than 1 million cases of brain damage over four decades of intensive use in the mentally ill. If a drug is so dangerous that its continued use is unjustified, as in the case of phenformin, a drug catastrophe comes to a satisfactory end. If a defect is so simple that it can be corrected—like putting the salt back into infant formula—the outcome is even better. But in the case of neuroleptic drugs, the corrective action has been mostly to sweep the problem under the rug. For example, a leading psychiatry textbook assures young practitioners that neuroleptic drugs "are remarkably safe." A review of treatment for schizophrenia in the *New England Journal of Medicine* declares, "Adverse effects are rarely serious or irreversible."[37] "Remarkably safe agents," concludes the leading pharmacology text.[38] The very worst outcome of a drug catastrophe is to pretend that it does not exist.

The injuries from drug catastrophe can only be estimated, but the totals justify nationwide alarm. Drugs for irregular heartbeats caused more than 50,000 deaths from cardiac arrest and sudden death in just a few years' time. Several hundred thousand cases of abnormal sexual organs occurred in the children of mothers who were given DES while pregnant. It is likely that more than 1 million cases of brain damage have been caused by neuroleptic drugs. There are few activities of modern society capable of causing severe injury or death on this scale. Fewer still combine a danger of catastrophe with a steady death toll that claims approximately 100,000 lives a year and injures 1 million severely enough to warrant hospitalization. Millions more are injured during other hospital treatment or experience injuries severe enough to need outpatient medical treatment. When society takes risks such as these, it is important to take the most careful measure of the benefits of drugs—the subject of the next chapter.

CHAPTER FOUR

The Benefits of Drugs

ONE MONDAY NIGHT IN June 1992, Jesse Kinison of Washington, D.C., failed to take the second of two prescribed daily doses of his medication. It was a serious mistake. The human body can survive for only minutes without oxygen. It can operate for a few days without water—and perhaps a few weeks without food. In the spectrum of urgent and essential human needs, Jesse Kinison's medication came second only to oxygen. Kinison was the night manager of a Western-style Washington bar called Remington's. This meant he worked late and slept late, and in this case he missed still another dose of medicine. By 10 A.M., he realized he was in big trouble. He called a friend, Denny, and said he needed to go to the hospital right away.

As Kinison stepped outside his apartment near the U.S. Capitol, he already had a sense of being detached from normal events on this planet. Everything around him seemed to be illuminated with unusually bright, white light. He had lost all normal sense of space and time. He asked his friend Denny if he also noticed this. Denny didn't see anything unusual, but noted Kinison was slurring his words. Things looked even worse by the time Kinison reached the emergency room of Georgetown University Hospital. The emergency room staff took a quick blood test and concluded he was probably not going to make it. His blood sugar was so high it was off the scale.

Jesse Kinison had failed to take two consecutive doses of a medicine essential to his survival. The drug was insulin. In examining the benefits of drugs, insulin makes a useful starting point because it is one of the most beneficial drugs ever discovered. In the United States alone, it daily keeps 500,000 people alive who would otherwise die.[1] Kinison survived. Given an emergency injection of insulin, he felt fine just six hours later. His failure to take the two prescribed injections was neither foolish nor negligent. He made a reasonable but erroneous guess about what he ought to do in an unusual situation. In juvenile-onset diabetes, the body loses its ability to manufacture any insulin. However, the injections of insulin must be carefully matched to food intake or else dangerously high or low blood-sugar levels will result. Because of a sore and unusually swollen throat, Kinison was eating almost nothing. So it seemed logical to cut back the insulin. Fortunately, he lived to tell about it.

If all drugs were as beneficial as insulin, then deciding whether to approve or take a new drug would be elementary. Insulin saved the life of the very first patient who received it. Not only are the benefits of insulin easy to document, the decision whether to take the drug is elementary indeed. You could take the drug—regardless of any adverse effects it might have. Or you could die.

However, among the 3,200 drugs in the armamentarium of modern medicine, only a handful have benefits of similar simplicity and magnitude.[2] These include drugs for general anesthesia, cyclosporine to prevent organ transplant rejection, and penicillin for meningococcal meningitis. In each case, the effects are lifesaving or very large; the benefits can be documented by simple observation within a short time. It takes only a few patients to demonstrate convincingly the medical benefit. The effects occur in most if not all of the patients treated.

At the other end of the scale, many widely used drugs have very small effect, or benefits occur in only a few of those treated. For example, consider the benefits of the drugs given to treat people with mild high blood pressure. Each year they prevent a stroke or heart attack in fewer than 2 of every 1,000 people who take them.[3] That means 99.8 percent of the people who took the medication faithfully every day of the year received no tangible benefit. The first drug for Alzheimers'—Cognex—produced a barely measurable 2-point gain on memory test scores. However, the observing physicians were unable to detect any overall improvement in careful periodic evaluations.[4] When the benefits are small or rare, even skilled physicians cannot reliably judge the effect of treatment. Drug benefits span the entire spectrum—from helping almost 100 percent of those treated to less than 1 percent.

Drugs with small benefits raise a host of important questions that simply do not arise with near miracle drugs. The effects—while real—may not be worth the cost. For example, Cognex costs about $1,700 a year.[5] Most important of all, since all drugs have adverse effects, a drug with small benefits can easily do more harm than good. (In the case of Cognex, 21 percent of patients showed substantial evidence of liver damage.)[6] In debates about approving new drugs, the issues are more likely to involve questions of efficacy—or benefits—than dangers or risks.[7] The pharmaceutical industry constantly pressures the FDA not so much to approve dangerous drugs but to be a more lenient judge of the benefits. It turns out that accurately judging the benefits of drugs is as difficult as measuring their risks. Worse yet, without scientific measures, both doctors and patients are likely to misjudge the benefits of drugs, believing that they work better than they do. These are some of the reasons.

The body's own remarkable capacity to heal itself greatly complicates the job of judging the benefits of drugs. In rare cases, people spontaneously recover from the most dire illnesses. The modern age of scientific medicine has not ended the reports of seemingly miraculous cures; if anything, such accounts about spontaneous remission of cancers and other remarkable recoveries have become a staple of popular health writing. Consider these examples:

The essayist and magazine editor Norman Cousins is hospitalized with a mysterious inflammatory disease that attacks the back, hip, shoulder, ribs, and jaw. Repelled at what he regards as the degrading and dehumanizing hospital environment, he checks himself out. Instead, he sits in a darkened room giggling and laughing at reel after reel of old Marx Brothers comedies. Inexplicably, he recovers.[8]

A molecular biologist named Alan Kapuler is diagnosed with cancer of the lymphatic system, with more than thirty abnormal nodes detected in a CT scan. He rejects chemotherapy as too toxic and self-prescribes a diet of brown rice, beans, sea vegetables, and other plant matter. He rejects meat, milk, sugar, oil, fruit, salads, and dietary supplements. Nine months later, the swollen lymph nodes are gone. Three years later, they recur, and this time he checks into a Mexican clinic that prescribes an herbal tonic but allows many more foods—except pork, tomatoes, and vinegar. Again he recovers.[9]

In 1952, four-year-old Ann O'Neil of Baltimore lay dying of leukemia. She had received the last rites. Her aunt had already made a yellow burial gown. Her parents took her to the cemetery, while still alive, and laid her on the grave of Mother Elizabeth Seton, founder of the Catholic order of the Sisters of

Charity. As the rain fell, O'Neil was surrounded by praying nuns. A few days later, a blood test revealed the leukemia had disappeared entirely. After Vatican investigators independently confirmed that her cancerous bone marrow had returned to normal, the Pope declared the event a miracle.[10]

Miraculous cures do occur. And if that individual happened to be taking a new or unusual drug, both patient and doctor tend to credit the drug. While such recoveries may be genuine, we cannot assume the drug was responsible. Testimonials from the miraculously cured patient have magnetic emotional appeal but are of no scientific value in establishing the benefits of drugs. Science requires that a predictable effect be observed under clearly stated conditions.

In *Remarkable Recovery*, a book about the spontaneous remission of cancer, the authors repeat a plausible and realistic rule of thumb: A practicing physician might witness one such inexplicable cure in a lifetime of medical practice.[11] This may be enough to spawn a whole literature of health books, but it would not demonstrate the effectiveness of any drug.

Doctors have another healing power that occurs much more frequently than miraculous cures and is more readily confused with the real benefits of drugs. Especially in the hands of a caring doctor, the ritual of medical treatment somehow focuses the patient's mind and body to speed recovery. Something in the union between doctor and patient repeatedly produces results that cannot be explained by the medical treatment itself. This can be seen in the results of an experiment in which the patients got better even though the treatment could not possibly have worked.

In the decades before James Black discovered beta-blockers, a dubious surgical operation was frequently performed to stop the chest pains of heart disease. In the chest are two small arteries that lie near the heart but do not supply it with blood. They are called the internal mammary arteries. In the early

1950s, a relatively simple and popular surgical procedure involved tying a suture around each internal mammary artery to halt the blood flow. Since these arteries weren't connected to the heart, the logic of this procedure was dubious at best. Nevertheless, at least one-third of the patients reported that the surgery greatly reduced their chest pains. Surgeons could produce enthusiastic patients to testify about the dramatic benefits. In a famous experiment at the University of Washington in Seattle, researchers demonstrated similar results in an entirely fake operation.[12] Patients were wheeled into the operating room, a small incision made, but no other surgery performed. Nevertheless, improvement was just as frequent in those who got the sham procedure as in those who actually received surgery.

This creates a special problem in judging the benefits of drugs. Not only was this treatment ineffective, but also the doctor and patient were sincerely—and sometimes passionately—convinced it worked. The only genuine beneficial effect came from the caring ritual of medical treatment. Such misleading testimonials have convinced even experienced medical professionals who should have known better. In judging the benefits of drugs, it is dangerous to be similarly fooled by the otherwise valuable effects of a caring doctor. In one famous medical essay, this placebo power was called "the lie that heals."[13]

Still another trap lies in wait to confuse the search for effective drugs. In a wide array of medical disorders, the symptoms come in short, severe episodes followed by periods of improvement or remission. This pattern can be seen in epilepsy, Parkinson's disease, ulcers, Alzheimer's, migraine headaches, hives, depression, anxiety, and multiple sclerosis. Especially when attended by the healing ritual of medical treatment, periods of improvement are often mistaken for an effect of a drug or other treatment.

Combine the natural fluctuations in disease with the real

healing power of a caring doctor and the effects are so large we cannot judge the benefits of drugs simply by counting the number who get better. Consider these results achieved in drug studies in which patients—without knowing it—were getting an inactive placebo for experimental purposes. The power of the placebo effect is stunning. In a ten-week study, a placebo eliminated panic attacks in 44 percent of patients.[14] In studies of hyperactive children, an average of 39 percent improved when given placebos.[15] In major depression, from 19 percent to 70 percent of the patients improved on placebos.[16] (The wide range of placebo effects in treating depression was mainly because of varying definitions of what constituted successful treatment.)

Dramatic placebo effects do not exist solely in the mind of the patients; they can be measured by laboratory tests. In an Australian study of blood pressure medication, researchers found that 25 percent of patients responded so well to a placebo that they no longer had high blood pressure.[17] One study of irregular heartbeats relied on a computer to analyze twenty-four-hour monitoring tapes. Irregular heartbeats were suppressed in 37 percent of those getting an inactive placebo.[18] In this case, the irregular heartbeats were too mild for the patients themselves to detect either before or after treatment. It took special cardiac monitors to identify the medical problem, and the effect of drug and placebo. The effects of inactive placebo drugs in heart failure are equally impressive. Notes one account, "Three months of treatment with a placebo produces a reduction in symptoms in 25 percent to 35 percent, an increase in cardiac output and a decrease in pulmonary wedge pressure, and an increase in exercise tolerance."[19] (In the case of these laboratory measurement examples, another effect is also involved called regression to the mean, but in such experiments it cannot be separated from the placebo effect.)

These are among the treacherous obstacles to judging the effectiveness of drugs. A single dramatic case can be genuine but completely misleading about the likely effects in a majority of patients. Because of the placebo effect, a doctor will see many patients improve—even if the prescribed drug is ineffective or harmful. Include the natural fluctuations of disease and we can expect from one-quarter to three-quarters to improve on a placebo. This shows why—even today—it would be easy to build a nationwide wave of enthusiasm for a quack remedy or untested drug. A miraculous recovery can provide a dramatic example for media coverage. The placebo effect will produce a legion of believing doctors and patients. Worse yet, these genuine effects are large enough to mask substantial harm. Patient deaths might be excused as a necessary price to pay for "a valuable new drug," or dismissed as an expected event in a sick-patient population. Ultimately, these obstacles explain why human society spent centuries actively searching for powerful medicines—but found so few until recent decades. No one could tell the difference between the beneficial and harmful drugs. Doctors and patients alike could be readily deceived by what they saw or experienced. The entire foundation of empirical science rested on the bedrock idea of systematic observation. Yet simple observation was not entirely reliable in the case of prescription drugs. It was not until the late 1940s that a valid method for measuring the benefits of drugs was first employed.

The symbol for justice is the blindfolded judge holding the scales on which the evidence can be weighed. In the randomized clinical trial, something quite close to that blindfolded judge was devised to establish the benefits of drugs. The first step in a valid test of the benefits of a drug is—in effect—to blindfold both the research doctor and the patient. The blindfold is achieved by manufacturing inert placebo pills that look absolutely identical to the real medication and packaging them in identical bottles. When the pills are dispensed, neither researcher nor patient knows whether the active drug is involved. Caring doctors and patients who want to get better are still involved. But some patients are going to get an active drug and some an inert placebo. That will be decided by random chance. Until the trial ends, and the results are tallied, neither the patients nor their doctors know who is taking the active drug. These are the key elements in the randomized clinical trial. Except for the rare drugs whose effects are so dramatic that they border on a miracle cure, the randomized clinical trial is the most reliable tool yet developed for judging the benefits and risks of drugs.

To observe the power—and often surprising findings—of the randomized clinical trial, consider a real-life scientific experiment with Prozac, the best-selling drug for depression. Before the trial begins, the investigators have already established that Prozac is a potent drug. It increases the concentration of a chemical called serotonin in the tiny gap between nerve cells in the brain and the central nervous system.[20] However, despite a clear biological effect, the drug may not have a net benefit. So the question is whether Prozac has a medical or health benefit, and the investigators must be specific. Will clearly measurable improvement be seen in a group of clinically depressed patients? The results that follow are expressed in simple round numbers but are actually taken from one of Eli Lilly's own published clinical trials of Prozac.[21]

The first step in a well-controlled trial is to recruit a group of patients who need treatment. If some of the subjects aren't truly sick or have some other medical problem, they probably won't benefit from an effective drug. In this case, we will recruit 200 patients who have been diagnosed by a psychiatrist with the disorder called "major clinical depression." This condition has a relatively precise definition.[22] The person must have symptoms such as being in a depressed mood most of the day for two weeks, or be contemplating suicide or experiencing feelings of worthlessness or inappropriate guilt. To qualify as major clinical depression, there must be present at least five of the nine such items on a list of symptoms. We will be more confident if several doctors in different locations helped recruit and treat the 200 patients. The annals of medicine are filled with accounts of a pioneering doctor reporting impressive results with a new treatment. However, other physicians were unable to reproduce the impressive results. It has never been clear whether these special doctors who get remarkable cures were selecting patients likely to improve anyway, had some gift for touching the mind of the patient that average physicians might lack, or were just quacks. In any case, we want to document the effects of a pill, not measure the talents of a physician.

Next, the 200 patients are randomly assigned to receive either Prozac or a pill of identical size and shape that is a harmless placebo. On the average, this results in about half the patients being assigned to the treatment group and half to placebo. Until the trial is over, neither the doctors nor the depressed patients know who is getting which. Assigning similar patients at random to receive an active drug or a placebo normally insures the two groups are almost exactly comparable. This means in both groups the severity of depression will be similar, as will be the average age, gender, and overall medical condition.

The experiment is still not ready to begin. Researchers must define in advance the medical result that the drug is expected to produce. At this moment, the art of medicine finally becomes a science. The researcher must know enough about the drug to state in writing an explicit prediction of the medical effects of the drug. For this test of Prozac, psychiatrists will evaluate each potential patient for depression, rating them on a severity scale with scores ranging from 0 to 52. Only those with a depression severe enough to score 20 or higher will be allowed into the experiment. Treatment will be counted as beneficial if the severity of depression is reduced by 50 percent or more on this scale. Although not a cure, it is a reasonable definition of "marked improvement."

After five weeks, the results are tallied. This was the actual result (in round numbers) from Eli Lilly's real clinical trial. Of the 100 patients, 38 showed "marked improvement" according to the definition. The remaining 62 had no benefit, dropped out because they couldn't tolerate the drug, or had a smaller benefit that didn't qualify as "marked." Although not a miracle cure, a marked improvement in 38 of 100 depressed patients sounds like a respectable result. But how about the patients getting the inactive placebo? In this untreated group, 19 of 100 showed marked improvement, getting better without any active drug. Since we don't want to credit the drug for patients who would have gotten better anyway, we subtract the placebo group to get the net effect: the drug appeared to be responsible for helping 19 of 100 patients treated.

The benefits of Prozac are, at best, modest. One research group at the University of Utah, finding similar effects in a separate clinical trial, concluded, "Although [Prozac] appeared to be an effective antidepressant in this investigation, the question arises whether it is a valuable addition to the antidepressant armamentarium."[23] In published studies and textbooks, much higher success rates would be repeatedly claimed for Prozac and similar drugs for depression. A common claim is that such drugs benefit about two-third of the patients. The more impressive claim is achieved by the dubious and selective use of statistics. First, the investigators forget about the 20 percent or more who dropped out. Second, the placebo effect—another 20 percent—is ignored and counted as a benefit of the drug. However, one clinical trial does not provide a complete evaluation of antidepressants. In many later clinical trials of other drugs for depression, benefits were even smaller, and sometimes not observed at all. [24] But despite the passionate Prozac testimonials seen in news media accounts and some books, the clinical trial provides the first piece of hard evidence on which to build a realistic overall picture of the drug.

At one extreme is a near miracle drug—insulin—in which nearly 100 of every 100 patients got lifesaving benefits. In the second case, Prozac, just 19 of 100 patients improved markedly, a result in the middle range of possible benefits, possibly below average. Much can be learned by looking at the other extreme— a drug with documented benefits so small that they lie near the threshold of what can be practically measured. Pravachol, the most effective cholesterol-lowering drug yet tested, is an excellent example.

Bristol-Myers Squibb sponsored a randomized clinical trial in Scotland to establish the tangible health benefits of Pravachol. The experiment had similar structure and blindfolding rules as that for Prozac. Even before the experiment began, Pravachol had a well-characterized biological effect—it lowered cholesterol levels. Virtually all modern receptor-based drugs have important biological effects—the question is whether making these changes in the body's control system improves health or prolongs life. As the rules of good science require, the investigators had to define what specific health benefit Pravachol was expected to achieve. In this case, they predicted that Pravachol would prevent heart attacks. Because heart attacks can be fatal about 10 percent of the time, the researchers also hoped to reduce the number of total deaths. Tracking deaths provides another important safety check. If a drug had serious adverse effects the investigators didn't even suspect, it could show up in unexpected patient deaths in the treatment group.

The trial was a great success and the predicted health benefits were achieved. However, heart attack or death was prevented in just 5 out of 1,000 men treated for a year. The other 995 got no tangible benefit. Over the entire five-year course of the Pravachol trial, only 2.4 percent benefited. To document credibly such a small effect, Bristol-Myers was forced to conduct a very lengthy clinical trial costing millions of dollars. It sponsored cholesterol tests for 160,000 men in west Scotland to locate 6,595 subjects with suitably high cholesterol levels—averaging 275 milligrams per deciliter (mg/dl). The recruited subjects had to take the medication—or a placebo—for five years. When drug companies run advertisements highlighting the millions of dollars they must spend to get a new drug to market, they do not usually explain one of the key reasons: When the effect is extremely small, it takes many years and requires thousands of participants and millions of dollars to measure such a small difference reliably. The five-year Pravachol results also reveal why so few benefited from treatment:

STATUS	PRAVACHOL	PLACEBO
Healthy	92.5%	89.9%
Heart attack	4.3%	6.2%
Died	3.2%	4.0%

As the table shows, 90 percent of the participants would have remained healthy whether treated or not. In promoting the drug, the manufacturer managed to find a way to state these small benefits in impressive terms. Bristol-Myers claims a dramatic 30 percent reduction in the risk of heart attack. The claim is technically correct—4.3 percent versus 6.2 percent is a 30 percent different. But such figures conceal the small effect of the drug.

The difference between the benefit profiles of insulin and Pravachol is striking for two reasons. Compared to juvenile-onset diabetes, having high cholesterol isn't nearly as dangerous a medical condition. Without insulin, every single patient will die in a few weeks' time. But even with Pravachol, 90 percent of the placebo group were still healthy five years later. (In fact, among men with high cholesterol the overall death rate is only a little higher than those with average cholesterol.)[25] Also, Pravachol prevented only about one-third of the heart attacks that occurred. Insulin was effective in virtually every case. The benefits of drugs for mild high blood pressure are of similar small size for the same reasons. They are effective in preventing about 40 percent of the strokes that would otherwise occur. But strokes are so rare in middle-aged persons that only about 2 out of 1,000 treated patients benefit in one year's time. Benefits are similarly modest for women who take estrogen to prevent hip and wrist fractures from calcium loss. (Estrogen has other risks and benefits that will be addressed later.)

Just because some drugs benefit only a small minority of those treated doesn't mean they are bad drugs, dangerous drugs, or should be avoided. Especially with drugs intended to prevent events such as heart attack or stroke, benefit rates are very low because it is hard to identify which patients really need the drug; as a result, thousands are treated who would have stayed healthy anyway. But even when a very small benefit is measured, some well-trained doctors declare a drug "is effective" and then prescribe it widely, forgetting about how few people will actually be helped. However, effectiveness is like having money in your pocket. The prudent will ask not only whether they have cash on hand, but how much.

The randomized clinical trial has another great power that reaches beyond an honest and practical measure of a drug's benefits. It also has the capacity to expose medical miscalculations about drug treatment that may endanger thousands of lives. The widely hailed antioxidant called beta-carotene provides an excellent case in point. A respectable but unproven theory holds that both cancer and the aging process may result from a dangerous form of oxygen inside human cells called free radicals. In this theory, some oxygen molecules are capable of triggering destructive chain reactions inside cells. Antioxidants are supposed to neutralize this danger. Many health advocates embraced beta-carotene because it was a "natural" antioxidant found in many fruits and vegetables and therefore ought to be free of health hazards. Even the National Cancer Institute jumped on the beta-carotene bandwagon, declaring, "A large body of epidemiological evidence indicates that cancer incidence is reduced as consumption of dietary vitamin A or its precursor, beta-carotene, found in dark green and yellow vegetables and fruits, increases."[26] The National Cancer Institute limited its recommendations to urging greater consumption of fruit and vegetables. However, many in the world of health advocacy concluded that if getting a little beta-carotene in vegetables seemed to be beneficial, then taking a vitamin supplement containing more of the chemical ought to be even better. The lack of clinical-trial evidence that taking this chemical was beneficial did not prevent many health advocates from recommending it. It was featured in best-selling health books such as *Life Extension and Spontaneous Healing*.[27] Such advice was featured in more mainstream medical publications, such as the *Wellness Letter* of the University of California at Berkeley.[28] The scientific advisory panel of the Alliance for Aging Research urged the government to include beta-carotene as a recommended daily vitamin.[29] As a result, millions of bottles of beta-carotene supplements were sold and consumed. Millions of people increased their vegetable consumption to get the beta-carotene.

In April of 1994, the first randomized clinical trial of beta-carotene was completed in Finland. Long after millions of people were taking beta-carotene, medical science was finally getting around to putting this interesting theory to the only valid scientific test—a randomized clinical trial. However, testing beta-carotene raised even more practical problems than testing Pravachol. Since cancer is a rarer event than a heart attack, it meant recruiting not merely thousands but tens of thousands of participants and observing them for five to eight years. Even then, given the small expected benefit, researchers had to limit the experiment to the highest-risk cancer population they could find: male cigarette smokers. Although the expected benefits were going to be quite small, a carefully designed, well-controlled trial would finally established that such benefits in fact existed.

The public and the scientific world were shocked at the results. The Finnish study showed that if taking beta-carotene had any effect, it was to increase the risk of lung cancer and death. However, the total effect, although harmful, was also very small. The net harm was just about 1 extra case of lung cancer for every 1,000 high-risk men who took it for one year. The embarrassed advocates of beta-carotene disbelieved the results. "Dangerously misleading," proclaimed Allan Smith of the University of California at Berkeley. "It borders on ludicrous to expect antioxidants to reduce cancer risk in six years of follow-up."[30] Even if one agreed with Smith, then it is hardly worth bothering with a chemical agent that had benefits so minuscule that they could not be observed among 30,000 high-risk subjects followed for up to eight years. Two years later, a flood of studies rounded out the picture. The National Cancer Institute halted its own clinical trial of beta-carotene among high-risk smokers because of excess deaths among those treated. It also terminated a study among 10,000 doctors, finding neither harm nor benefit. In the doctors trial, the benefits or harm was so small that they were not apparent in this large but healthy group after ten years of continuous observation.

In this instance, randomized clinical trials saved the public and the health establishment from making a gross mistake.

Depending on how one wants to interpret the results, beta-carotene supplements are either harmful or have too little effect to bother about. Beta-carotene is a vitamin and not subject to the strict controls applied to the potentially more dangerous prescription drugs. But the issues and the results were the same.

This leads to one of the central lessons of this chapter: Establishing the tangible health benefits of drugs protects the public from major dangers that no one anticipated or expected. And some doctors and patients still embrace drugs based on testimonials rather than evidence. Unfortunately, the mainstream medical establishment and the FDA accept drugs based on biological effect or a medical theory rather than clear evidence of a tangible health benefit from a randomized clinical trial. As a result, terrible mistakes are frequently revealed when clinical trials are finally completed—often after hundreds of thousands of people are already exposed to danger. A thyroid hormone used to lower cholesterol apparently caused heart attacks rather than prevented them—as medical theory assumed.[31] Tambocor, a drug that suppressed irregular heartbeats, caused cardiac arrest instead of preventing it.[32] Milrinone, a drug that increased the output of already weakened hearts, increased the risk of death. In each of these cases, the drugs had well-documented biological effects supported by credible medical theory. But when a clinical trial tested for a genuine health benefit, these drugs proved to be harmful.

A clinical trial, then, is the only reliable tool for separating beneficial drugs from harmful ones, the test that differentiates a reliable cure from a rare but remarkable recovery, and distinguishes the chemical effect from the real but less tangible benefits of a caring physician. The stories about prescription drugs throughout this book will show that the centuries-old tendency to be foolishly optimistic about the benefits of drugs is often a more serious problem than ignorance about their dangers. These last two chapters have focused on the tangible, measurable effects of drugs, both harmful and beneficial. The next chapters examine potentially harmful drug effects that are difficult to measure but are of no less importance than the effects that are clear and tangible.

CHAPTER FIVE

Drugs and Behavior

THE FIRST THING Diane Ayres noticed was that her left arm had suddenly become numb. A few hours earlier, she had taken the first dose of Floxin, a broad-spectrum antibiotic. Then her vision got cloudy. Next, she became confused. Ayres, who worked at home, got lost in her own office; she was also unable to figure out how to turn off her own computer. Then she started to shake uncontrollably. Thinking she might be dying, she called her husband, Stephen Fried, and told him something was wrong. By the time he got home, he found her in the closet, uncertain where she was, looking for a white blouse, which was located an inch from her hand. By the time she reached the emergency room, her pupils were fixed and dilated and she was unable to speak in complete sentences.[1]

The manufacturer's disclosure statement notes that Floxin "may also cause central nervous system stimulation which may lead to: tremors, restlessness/agitation, nervousness/anxiety, light-headedness, confusion, hallucinations, paranoia and depression, nightmares, insomnia, and rarely suicidal thoughts or acts. These reactions may occur following the first dose."[2]

Mrs. A. was one of those women who was never satisfied with herself. A marriage and three children had done little or nothing to reduce her sense of inadequacy, which often triggered long bouts of crying. Her doctor prescribed Prozac, and after two weeks she responded well. As with many people who take this powerful stimulant, Mrs. A. felt energized and newly self-confident. She stopped crying. Two weeks later, she was delivered in handcuffs to the psychiatric ward of a nearby hospital. For the first time in her life, she had experienced a terrifying condition called a manic attack. She hardly ate or slept. This normally quiet and shy person became expansive and loquacious, spending excessively at garage sales. Then things got worse. She broke into a neighbor's house. She accused her minister of committing murder. And she finally ended up in handcuffs after attacking three policemen. This manic psychotic behavior disappeared soon after she stopped taking Prozac, although she was hospitalized for several weeks. In the next eight months, without Prozac, she had no further manic attacks.[3]

Eli Lilly, manufacturer of Prozac, says, "During premarketing testing, hypomania or mania occurred in approximately 1% of fluoxetine [Prozac] treated patients."[4] (Hypomania is a less severe form of elevated mood that typically doesn't require hospitalization.) In March of 1996, according to Eli Lilly, 754,000 new prescriptions were written for Prozac.[5] If episodes appear at about the rate Lilly reported in drug testing, then that would amount to 7,500 cases among new Prozac patients in a single month. However, there is simply no way of knowing how many cases of mania—moderate or severe—are being triggered by antidepressant drugs.

For many years Ilo Marie Grundberg of Salt Lake City had cared for her mother, Mildred Coates. But at age eighty-three, and suffering memory loss from Alzheimer's, she had become an ever greater mental and physical burden to her daughter, who had difficulty sleeping and was prescribed the popular sleep medication Halcion in the then recommended dose of 0.5 milligram. However, the normally quiet and law-abiding Grundberg was not told that Halcion was capable of causing "hallucinations, delusions, aggressiveness, falling, somnambulism, syncope, inappropriate behavior, and other adverse behavioral effects." On June 19, 1988, Marie Grundberg exploded in a murderous rage and fired eight bullets into her peacefully sleeping mother, leaving a birthday card tucked into her hand. In the aftermath of this horrible tragedy, Grundberg won two legal victories. She was indicted for manslaughter, but the charges were dropped after the judge allowed Grundberg's defense that she was involuntarily intoxicated by Halcion. She later sued Upjohn for $21 million in damages and won a settlement of undisclosed size.[6] By 1987, Upjohn had received reports of twenty-four cases of murder, attempted murder, or threat of physical attack associated with Halcion.[7]

We know that chemicals influence human behavior. With high blood levels of alcohol, some people will commit acts too horrible to contemplate when cold sober. Policemen and emergency medical workers have coped with people so crazed on amphetamines, crack cocaine, or hallucinogens that it is hard to describe such behavior as rational or even "human." The growing array of chemicals that influence human behavior clashes directly with long-standing doctrines woven deeply into the fabric of society. Our moral and legal tradition depends on the central idea that we each are responsible for our acts. Without that responsibility, the moral basis for trial and punishment for crimes is undermined. However, the desire to make society work—and to take the stern view of individual responsibility—should not lead to denying the powerful but often unexpected effects of prescription drugs on behavior.

An ever growing fraction of the population routinely takes powerful prescription drugs that rearrange the electrochemical circuits through which all human feelings, thought, and behavior flow. A growing ability to identify, stimulate, or block chemical receptors that are involved in behavior has not been accompanied by an adequate grasp of how the whole system works. Most of what is known involves crude extremes. If the brain cells that secrete a chemical neurotransmitter called dopamine are destroyed, the result is a frozen zombie who cannot move muscles voluntarily. However, if dopamine receptors are stimulated with an agonist drug such as LSD, the result is bizarre perceptions and actions. Even less is known about serotonin. Still, we are treated to discourses about the "clean effects" of Prozac, Paxil, and Zoloft because they are seemingly targeted on serotonin receptors in the brain rather than several different neurotransmitters. But the functional purpose of serotonin neurotransmitters remains largely unknown. In terms of ability to relieve clinical depression, the antidepressants produce similar results regardless of the neurotransmitters they are presumed to affect.[8] It is as though researchers have learned the function of some of the transistors in a radio but still don't understand why it is playing soft rock music instead of the baseball game. Change the transistor in an unmapped behavioral circuit, and it is not surprising to observe unexpected and unwanted results at least some of the time. In addition to prescription drugs that are intended to alter feeling and behavior, there are hundreds more that produce unintended and unwanted adverse effects on behavior. To get a sense of the scope of effects and the number of drugs implicated, consider this list of adverse effects, culled from the disclosure labels of approved drugs. After each adverse effect, the number of drugs associated with it appears in parentheses:

Aggression (19)

Agitation (143)

Agoraphobia (1)

Amnesia (48)

Amnesia, traveler's (1)

Anger (4)

Anorexia (386)

Anxiety (239)

Anxiety, paradoxical (38)

Aphonia (3)

Argumentativeness (1)

Asthenia (399)

Awareness, altered (3)

Awareness, heightened (3)

Behavior, hypochondriacal (1)

Behavior, inappropriate (9)

Behavior, violent (1)

Behavioral changes (20)

Behavioral deterioration (2)

Blackout spells (6)

Character changes (1)

Claustrophobia (2)

Confusion (314)

Confusion, mental (314)

Confusion, nocturnal (2)

Confusional state (314)

Coordination difficulty (41)

CNA (central nervous system) stimulation (36)

CNS stimulation, paradoxical (5)

Cognitive dysfunction (12)

Combativeness (2)

Coordination, disturbed (41)

Coordination, impaired (41)

Coordination, lack of (173)

Crying (16)

Delirium (27)

Delusions (38)

Dementia (11)

Depersonalization (28)

Depression (242)

Depression, aggravation of (3)

Depression, mental (150)

Depression, mood (150)

Depression, psychotic (2)

Depressive reactions (2)

Despondency (1)

Disorientation (84)

Disorientation, place (17)

Disorientation, time (17)

Disturbances, emotional (16)

Dreaming abnormalities (84)

Dysphoria (204)

Elation (1)

Emotional disturbances (16)

Emotional lability (67)

Energy, high (6)

Energy, loss of (11)

Excitability (111)

Excitement, paradoxical (14)

Euphoria (138)

Fear (29)

Floating feeling (7)

Feeling intoxicated (7)

Feeling shaky (4)

Feeling strange (4)

Feeling drugged (2)

Giddiness (692)

Hallucinations (204)

Hallucinations, auditory (4)

Hallucinations, hypnagogic (1)

Hallucinations, visual (10)

Hostility (20)

Hyperirritability (5)

Hyperactivity (27)

Hypomania (19)

Hysteria (22)

Idiosyncrasy (17)

Impulse control, impaired (1)

Indecisiveness (1)

Insomnia (418)

Insomnia, early morning (1)

Intoxication, chronic (2)

Irritability (109)

Jitteriness (10)

Lassitude (27)

Laughing, easy (1)

Listlessness (4)

Malaise (229)

Manic behavior (35)

Memory impairment (36)

Memory loss, short-term (34)

Mental clouding (13)

Mental confusion (314)

Mental depression (150)

Mental perception, altered (1)

Mental performance, impairment (107)

Mental slowness (3)

Mental status, altered (23)

Moaning (1)

Mood changes (58)

Motor and phonic tics, exacerbations (2)

Motor disturbances, reversible involuntary (1)

Motor skills, impairment (27)

Muscular disturbances (10)

Nervousness (325)

Night terrors (1)

Nightmares (58)

Overstimulation (21)

Paranoia (38)

Personality changes (26)

Psychoses (108)

Psychoses, aggravation (21)

Psychoses, toxic (11)

Psychosis, activation (7)

Psychosis, overt (1)

Psychosis, paranoid (1)

Psychotic episodes (111)

Rage (6)

Retardation, psychomotor (3)

Schizophrenia, precipitation (2)

Screaming, excessive (1)

Sedation (95)

Sleep disturbances (64)

Sleepiness (492)

Sleeplessness (418)

Speech, bulbar type (1)

Speech difficulties (7)	Suicidal ideation (32)
Speech disturbances (37)	Suicide, attempt of (22)
Speech, incoherent (3)	Talkativeness (7)
Speech, slurring (37)	Thinking abnormality (45)
Self-deprecation (1)	Trembling (28)
Sluggishness (6)	Unsteadiness (7)
Sociopathy (4)	Weakness (399)
Stupor (32)	Yawning (18)

Unwanted effects on mood and behavior are most common among drugs targeted on receptors in the brain or central nervous system, especially sedatives, tranquilizers, antidepressants, and neuroleptic drugs for severe mental illness. But they are also seen in a wide array of other agents, notably some antibiotics, antihistamines, blood pressure drugs, diet pills, and drugs for asthma and epilepsy. The severity of the effect also spans the entire spectrum. It seems silly for a manufacturer to list "crying" as an adverse effect of several immunizations for infants. At the other extreme, drugs trigger frightening aberrations such as suicide attempts, manic attacks, and outright psychotic and sociopathic behavior. Such behaviors usually require confinement in a mental health facility, the stigma of a major mental illness, and often a prescription for dangerous and powerful neuroleptic drugs that even when working as intended suppress feeling and behavior.

Scanning the list for the adverse effects linked to very large numbers of drugs, an obvious pattern emerges. Drugs frequently depress the central nervous system. So we find 399 listed drugs that may cause asthenia, the medical term that means "depleted vitality." Another 242 have been blamed for outright depression, and an additional 229 are linked to malaise. The opposite effect—overstimulating the system is also common. So the list includes 239 drugs associated with anxiety as an adverse effect, and another 325 that may cause nervousness, 143 associated with agitation, and 111 linked to excitability.

In many cases, people stop taking medication that makes them too excited or too depressed. However, sometimes people don't realize a drug is behind a bout of depression, anxiety, or excitement. Others don't know that sometimes a switch to another drug takes care of the problem. To get some medical benefits—for example, to prevent epileptic seizures, or reduce the most severe pain—many people will tolerate major adverse effects. For example, one woman, overstimulated by her new diet pills, said, "I've still got a couple of rooms to clean, but then what? I feel like I've had WAY too much caffeine." Mostly, the adverse effects stop when the person stops taking the drug.

A third group of drugs may impair memory and thought. Mental confusion can result from 314 drugs, and another 107 cause impaired mental performance. At least 36 drugs are linked to memory impairment, and another 34 list short-term memory loss as an adverse effect. Other drugs may cause black-out spells, altered mental status, impaired motor skills, or incoherent speech. These effects can be more treacherous because sometimes the individual remains unaware of the impairment, let alone the cause.

Our greatest concern should be reserved for the drugs that may cause behavior so extreme that long-standing relationships are destroyed or violence occurs. These more severe reported drug effects include rage, aggression, violent behavior, mania, psychotic episodes, and thoughts of, or attempts at, suicide. At least 226 drugs list an association with these severe effects. The true cost of these terrible episodes is that individuals are often unable to resume, unchanged, the lives they had before. The following report gives you the flavor of such tragedies. This story is from an Internet support group for people using diet drugs, especially "fen/phen," the nickname for the combination of fenfluramine and phentermine.*

Hello everybody.
I just wanted to share this with you. I think that the people taking fen/phen and their families should all know about this. My husband and I went on a fen/phen program. It was great, the pounds flew off. Other than the dry mouth, and some difficulty falling to sleep, everything seemed great. As time went on, I noticed my husband started to become more irritable, and after carefully considering my own behavior I realized that I had too. The women out there can relate to it feeling like a moderate but extended bout of PMS. In the meantime, our doctor became concerned about the side effects of fenfluramine, and didn't think it was worth the risk of developing lung disease. Although he was an enthusiastic proponent of fen before, he stopped prescribing it. He continued to prescribe the phentermine. I stopped taking both because I was skeptical of the benefits of phen alone.

But my husband continued, in fact the doctor increased his dose as the food cravings started coming back. My husband became *very* irritable. He would fly off the handle at the least provocation. Everyone and everything made him angry. I explained this to the doctor, and he agreed that, yes, this could happen. My husband did not want to stop the phentermine, he only had 20 pounds to reach his goal. The doctor put him on Paxil (an SSRI in the same family as Prozac) to control the irritability. The Paxil was wonderful . . . at first. After a few weeks, around ten to twelve hours after his dose he would be more tense and irritable than ever. My husband also has had to begin taking testosterone shots every two weeks. Yesterday he had his shot.

Last night he flew into a rage, and became suicidal. I had to

* In the fall of 1997, fenfluramine was withdrawn because of adverse effects on heart valves.

call the police, and he was arrested. Our marriage is probably finished now. I don't believe that he will ever forgive me. We were one of those sickening couples who were totally devoted to each other, working together, playing together, and missing each other if we spent more than a few hours apart. We were each other's best friends. Yes, we had arguments, but we also loved each other intensely. Now it's all over. I am telling you this because, although many people have taken these medications without any major problems, some people will be affected like my husband. It can start without the person even knowing it's happening. I don't think my husband even knows yet the huge difference in his personality. I wish I had my old life back, fat and all. Because now, I feel like I've lost everything.

> Good luck to you all,
> Cathy

A few days later, things had improved. Her husband was off diet drugs and tapering off the Paxil. He was also seeing a counselor. Any specific episode is likely to generate debate about what was really responsible. Was the doctor to blame for prescribing a high-powered psychostimulant, Paxil, to someone already anxious and irritable from taking another drug—phentermine—with stimulant properties? In truth, the disclosure label for Paxil alone lists enough behavioral adverse effects to account for the story:

NERVOUS SYSTEM:

Frequent: amnesia, CNA stimulation, concentration impaired, depression, emotional lability, vertigo; Infrequent: abnormal thinking, akinesia, alcohol abuse, ataxia, convulsion, depersonalization, hallucinations, hyperkinesia, hypertonia, incoordination, lack of emotion, manic reaction, paranoid reaction; Rare: abnormal electroencephalogram, abnormal gait, antisocial reaction, choreoathetosis, delirium, delusions, diplopia, drug dependence, dysarthria, dyskinesia, dystonia, euphoria, fasciculations, grand mal convulsion, hostility, hyperalgesia, hypokinesia, hysteria, libido increased, manic-depressive reaction, meningitis, myelitis, neuralgia, neuropathy, nystagmus, paralysis, psychosis, psychotic depression, reflexes increased, stupor, withdrawal syndrome.

Hallucinations (219 drugs) are another frequent adverse behavioral effect. They are associated with a wide array of drugs—painkillers, antibiotics, blood pressure drugs, antidepressants, tranquilizers, and drugs for epilepsy, irregular heart rhythms, and migraine headaches. As the following example suggests, even a fairly mild case can be alarming.

In the summer of 1994 Barbara Wilkes of Washington, D.C., came home with two prescriptions for her persistent bronchitis. One was an antibiotic. The other was for the mildest narcotic drug in widespread use: prescription cough syrup with codeine. On Friday night, she had taken the second of two prescribed doses of cough syrup and lay down on the couch of her home in northwest Washington. Soon she was looking out the window of her thoroughly landlocked house and, surprisingly, was seeing the ocean and a beach. "I wanted to go to the beach. I could feel the ocean," she said. "I insisted to my roommate, Laurie, that we should go swimming. I wouldn't drop it. This conversation persisted for fifteen minutes. It finally ended when Laurie said to go to sleep and we would go swimming tomorrow. At that I did go to sleep, but I dreamed about the ocean. When I woke up, I was very scared. My heart was pounding. It shook me up. Laurie was so worried she made me sleep in her room."

The examples for this chapter were selected for their simplicity and their clarity. Either they occurred among otherwise healthy, reasonably well-adjusted people or the behavior involved was so extreme and so unprecedented that a neutral observer is willing to consider a drug as a likely suspect. Unfortunately, the evidence is not so crisp in a large majority of cases. An individual, soon after starting a new prescription, becomes depressed, but like so many of us, has been depressed before. If the drug is not one of the most familiar suspects—such as beta-blockers—neither a busy physician nor an unskeptical consumer is likely to link the depression to the drug. Other than knowing an awesome number of drugs may be involved, we can't even venture to guess how many cases might occur each year. But the label disclosure statement that Prozac and other antidepressant drugs might activate mania or hypomania in 1 percent of patients is frightening indeed. Behavioral effects rank among the most severe disabling injuries caused by prescription drugs. But the cases are not treated, identified, counted, or analyzed for lessons about how to identify those who might be the most vulnerable or otherwise at high risk.

To make matters worse, the most serious cases of bizarre, harmful behavior probably occur in patient populations where these effects are most likely to be dismissed—those with a previous medical history of psychological problems. A simple analogy illustrates the problem. If a drug damages the liver, the first cases might well be seen among patients with a vulnerable liver already damaged by alcohol abuse. Similarly, a summer storm is likely to claim an aging and vulnerable tree. In this situation, most people would still blame the storm. But given a patient with liver problems, the physician is more likely to blame new evidence of harm on the alcohol rather than on the drug. By a similar logic, many of the early reports of bizarre, suicidal, and other dangerous behavior among patients taking Xanax, Halcion, and Prozac were dismissed because many of the victims had been previously treated for psychiatric problems. Given a system already prone to ignoring the risks of drugs, the ambiguous problem of drug-induced behavior offers new opportunities for denial. However, as the next story illustrates, denial reaches new heights for the oldest and most pervasive behavioral adverse effect of prescription drugs.

Few moments in life are more terrible than the cold, unforgiving day when a person with a lifelong record of success realizes he has been completely and utterly defeated. Such a day arrived in the summer of 1995 for a Boston area doctor named Christopher Iliades.[9] The instrument of his defeat was a prescription drug called hydrocodone—a synthetic narcotic included in many popular cough syrups and pain remedies. The ashes of defeat were particularly bitter because Iliades believed he had already learned how to resist the siren's lure of addictive drugs.

Iliades, an ear, nose, and throat specialist, can still remember the day on which his journey to addiction began. He was suffering from a nasty sinus infection and facing a waiting room full of patients. Every year, pharmaceutical companies give each practicing doctor thousands of free drug samples, and Iliades was no exception. In this case, he had been left an entire case of a cough syrup that contained hydrocodone as the narcotic. It was called Tussenex. So he took a teaspoon of the cough syrup. Somewhere in his body a light went on. "It was a revelation," Iliades recalled, "like, 'Hello, where have you been all my life?'" He felt warm. He felt energized and eager to tackle the rest of his waiting room full of patients. The next time he had a headache or felt bad, he took the wonderful cough syrup instead of an aspirin. Within a matter of months, he found himself using it whenever he needed a boost to get through an unusually tough day at work. But he never used it on weekends. Then came the day when he finally figured out why he felt so lousy on the weekends. It was withdrawal symptoms for the hydrocodone. For the first time in his life, he found himself addicted to a drug.

This continued for nearly ten years. No one noticed anything. He liked the way the narcotic made him feel: relaxed, confident, and energetic. Then one day he confessed his problem to a state drug investigator who had come to interview him about the narcotics prescriptions he was writing for members of his family. He reported his problem to the Massachusetts Medical Society and entered a thirty-day inpatient treatment program. Withdrawal was difficult. "You have the feeling your whole body is shutting down. You're exhausted and nauseous, drenched with terrible sweats. Your muscles twitch and you get chills and headaches. It is like having the flu ten times over." He following up the treatment by joining in an outpatient therapy group. By confronting his drug addiction directly and openly, he was able to resume his medical practice while being monitored. All this unfolded according to the modern medical textbook approach to drug addiction and dependency. But four years later, Iliades would open another, darker chapter in the textbook of addiction.

One day, a patient with throat cancer arrived with a paper bag filled with pain medication, a collection from several different prescribing specialists over several months' time. Iliades selected the painkillers then appropriate for the patient. But he kept the bag and all the remaining pills. He told himself he was going to leave the bag in the garbage at the end of his office hours. But he didn't. He yielded to a bottle of his old friend, Tussenex. Next he told himself he would only take the medicine in the bag on unusual occasions. He began to ration the dwindling supply carefully. Then one day, no more narcotic medication was left in the bag. Because he was monitored, he could not write a prescription himself. So he lied to a colleague to get a prescription. But when he tried to fill this prescription for another person, a suspicious pharmacist challenged it. It was at that moment that Iliades realized he had been completely and utterly defeated by a commonly prescribed painkiller. One year later, he had completed a three-month special treatment program for health professionals and was working on a landscaping crew to make ends meet, hoping that his suspended medical license would soon be restored. But because of hydrocodone, his life would never again be the same.

The habit-forming property of drugs may be the oldest, most widespread, and among the most serious of all adverse effects. Every year, nearly 400,000 people visit the emergency room because of an overdose, dependency, or other urgent problem from illicit use of prescription drugs.[10] According to the leading federal household survey, 6 million people say in the last year they made "nonmedical" use of tranquilizers, sedatives, stimulants, or painkillers.[11] This is roughly twice as many as who said they used cocaine or heroin. However, the numbers dwindled to 2.5 million people when the survey researchers counted only those who said they used these prescription drugs illicitly in the past month—rather than a full year. In 1992, nearly 100,000 persons were hospitalized with a diagnosis of "poisoning" by psychologically active drugs, with 90 percent of the cases evenly divided between benzodiazepine tranquilizers and antidepressants. (This one adverse effect of drugs produces as many hospitalizations as do all auto accidents.)

It is a problem that has reached into the lives of some of the nation's most celebrated citizens. Two years after leaving the White House, Betty Ford was hospitalized for treatment of Valium drug dependence and for alcohol problems, a situation that had afflicted her for years.[12] Kitty Dukakis, wife of 1988 Democratic presidential nominee Michael Dukakis, revealed she was addicted for twenty-six years to amphetamines—initially taken to help control her weight.[13] And the chief justice of the Supreme Court, William Rehnquist, became dependent on Placidyl, a sleep medication.

Rehnquist was prescribed Placidyl because his sleep was interrupted by recurring back pain. He took the drug—recommended for only two weeks' continuous use—for nine years at up to three times the recommended dose.[14] Before he entered a Washington, D.C., hospital for detoxification, he was observed slurring words and appearing confused while hearing cases on the Supreme Court bench.

Because of technical problems and varying definitions, the national survey figures do not give a very accurate picture of the problems caused by addictive and habit-forming prescription drugs. Addiction to prescription drugs is often part of a more complex problem that includes alcohol, illegal street drugs, and suicide attempts and gestures. On the other hand, the addiction data barely touches on what is probably the typical prescription drug dependency case—cases like those of Christopher Iliades, Kitty Dukakis, William Rehnquist, and Betty Ford. For many years, they became gradually more dependent on a legally prescribed drug. They didn't go to an emergency room with an overdose. They didn't steal drugs or use them for recreation. Such cases must number in the hundreds of thousands—but we can only guess. All this evidence does show that addiction to prescription drugs is a very large problem involving a significant fraction of the adult population.

Most potentially addictive drugs make people feel good. Cocaine, Ritalin, and amphetamines are stimulants that make people feel energetic and confident and believe they are thinking especially clearly. Benzodiazepine tranquilizers and barbiturates make people feel relaxed, help them sleep better, and free them from anxious and nervous feelings. Heroin, codeine, hydrocodone, and other narcotic drugs not only relieve pain but create a warm, euphoric elevated mood. The more rapid and extreme the mood effects, the more likely that a drug will be, in the official terminology, "abused." Thus, injected heroin, snorted cocaine, or snorted Ritalin provide a mood change that is dramatic and has rapid onset. By contrast, an antidepressant drug such as Prozac takes weeks to achieve its effect—and is a poor candidate for the instant gratification typical of recreational use.

If mood elevation is the carrot of a potentially addictive drug, the combination of tolerance and withdrawal are the stick. Because the body makes chemical adjustments in the brain and central nervous system to tolerate the continued intrusion of psychoactive drugs, withdrawal symptoms can occur when the drug is abruptly removed. These symptoms including sweating, a rapid heartbeat, panic, anxiety, sleeplessness, hallucinations, agitation, jerking muscles, dizziness, delirium, increased sensitivity to light and sound, vomiting, diarrhea, fever, and seizures. Not only does the drug-dependent person want the pleasurable effects of the drug; when deprived of it, they suffer symptoms that range from alarming and unpleasant feelings to outright life-threatening events. Benzodiazepine tranquilizers are complex because individual responses vary, and some people develop tolerance to the drug's effects on sleep but not to its effects on anxiety, which persist at a stable dose.[15] Drugs that do not typically induce the desire for ever higher doses nevertheless produce a fearsome array of withdrawal symptoms when stopped. For example, Xanax can result in extremely difficult drug withdrawals requiring prolonged hospitalization of people who have never taken more than the prescribed dose.[16] In addition to these measurable reactions, many of these drugs induce a form of psychological dependence that may be without a basis in any physical symptoms. Some people who take tranquilizers or antidepressants believe they can't do without the drugs and refuse to give them up—even while taking their usual dose and therefore free of any physical withdrawal symptoms.

With barbiturates—drugs such as Seconal, Nembutal, and

Amytal—the carrot-and-stick effects come in a particularly lethal combination. The drugs depress the central nervous system in menacing sequential manner. Increasing doses cause relaxation, mild sedation, sleep, unconsciousness, coma, and death.[17] The lethal dose is about ten times the starting dose. However, tolerance occurs readily, leading some patients to increase the dose continuously to get the same effect on anxiety or sleep. In just two weeks' time, a 50 percent greater dose could be required to achieve the same effects. With each advancing month, users march closer and closer to the lethal dose. Trying to cut back triggers withdrawal symptoms of anxiety and insomnia. To add to the hazard, the other common depressant—alcohol—greatly increases the potentially lethal effects. As a result, thousands upon thousands of people have killed themselves with barbiturates. When Valium was introduced as the first major benzodiazepine tranquilizer, one major claim was its greater safety. Tolerance did not develop so quickly; it was more selective for anxiety and sleep without as large a depressing effect on the overall central nervous system, and the combination with alcohol was not quite so lethal. However, as use of tranquilizers exploded, overdose deaths became distressingly commonplace.

For reasons no one yet understands, the carrot and the stick of addiction drive some individuals more powerfully than others. Some may have a greater craving for the elevated mood, or experience a life that is filled with more anxiety, depression, or anguish. Some people may be affected by unusually sharp pains of withdrawal or develop tolerance more quickly, seeking ever greater amounts of the drug. Slowly but surely, it can take over a life. Individuals find they cannot cut down or discover their normal life priorities, which are distorted by desire for the drug. This is the first major way station in addiction, or "substance dependence" in the current official medical jargon.[18] It reaches a level described as "substance abuse" when the drug has so taken over life that jobs, marriage, family are compromised, or behavior occurs that leads to arrest or violence.[19]

Addiction may be unique among major adverse effects of drugs because society has had so many decades of experience wrestling with the problem. However, society appears to have learned little, repeating the same mistake time after time. More than a century ago, the panacea drug was opium. In the late nineteenth century, the United States was importing enough raw opium to provide fifty doses to every man, woman, and child in the country.[20] It was not until 1914 that the first narcotics control measures were enacted. In the same period that awareness was increasing about the hazards of opium, the next panacea drug—cocaine—was already gaining in popularity. Sigmund Freud waxed poetic about cocaine's properties; another physician, Conan Doyle, made it the drug of choice of the legendary fictional detective Sherlock Holmes.[21] Cocaine was the psychologically active ingredient in Coca-Cola—later to be replaced by caffeine.

The growing understanding of cocaine's dangers did little to restrain medical enthusiasm for the next addictive panacea drug—the amphetamines. By the mid 1950s, amphetamine drugs were being sold for multiple uses: anxiety, depression, obesity, fatigue, arthritis, and headaches. In the same period, more than 50 barbiturate drugs—with their special addiction and overdose dangers—were on the market and more than 2,500 had been synthesized. By the 1960s, amphetamines had become popular illicit drugs triggering violence and psychotic episodes. These experiences led to controls on amphetamines, barbiturates, and narcotics—but not to more careful scrutiny of the addiction potential of their replacements.

By that time Valium, Librium, and other benzodiazepine tranquilizers had become the panacea drugs of choice. They were advertised as safer than barbiturates, which proved to be at least partly true, and nonaddictive, which proved to be false. While most tranquilizers didn't produce a rapid high, some of them proved to have withdrawal problems as difficult as any known addictive drug.[22] The lessons on addiction learned form narcotics were ignored in 1957 when Eli Lilly introduced Darvon, a new painkiller. Even though it chemically resembled opium and morphine, it was advertised as free of the addiction dangers posed by codeine. By the late 1970s, Darvon was recognized as having addiction risks similar to codeine and the barbiturates, and more than 1,000 people died every year from overdoses.[23] However, in relieving pain it was no more effective than aspirin.[24]

A century's experience with addictive painkillers had little effect on the FDA, which in 1995 approved Ultram, a new painkiller touted (like Darvon) as more effective than aspirin without the addictive properties of opiates. In the rush to approve Ultram, the FDA did not delay approval of the drug while the manufacturer conducted studies of whether Ultram was addictive. Johnson & Johnson was allowed to do these studies after the commercial launch of the drug.[25] Only a year elapsed before the FDA had to require new warnings of Ultram's addiction dangers after receiving more than a hundred reports about addiction and overdose problems.[26] The current panacea drugs are the antidepressants—Prozac, Zoloft, and Paxil. If you listen to patients, they have similar—and apparently pronounced—withdrawal effects, making it difficult to stop treatment.

"I recently reduced my Paxil dosage," noted Michael Sharkey, a minister. "After three days, I was surprised—'shocked'—to feel electrical-type shocks zipping through my body several times per hour. At night, I had difficulty sleeping because I heard strange sounds which resembled the sound of an electronic buzz."

"After almost a year on Zoloft, I ran out of it," said William

Corson, "and I didn't get the prescription refilled. Three days later, I had the first grand mal seizure of my life. The days prior to it felt very much like little electric shocks going through my body."

Despite the nation's long history of underestimating drug dependence, tolerance, and withdrawal effect, Roerig, the manufacturer, declares, "Zoloft has not been systematically studied in animals or humans for its potential for abuse, tolerance or physical dependence." Prozac and Paxil have identically worded declarations of ignorance. Because these drugs take weeks to produce their mood effects, they are unlikely candidates for illicit street use for quick "highs." However, it is also clear many people have difficulty stopping antidepressants, and no manufacturer is likely to sponsor the research needed to find out just how difficult this may be, and how many people are affected.

Decades of experience now reveal a predictable cycle for these drugs that make people feel good. They are introduced with enthusiastic claims of the near miracles they accomplish. Disturbing reports of addiction, tolerance, withdrawal, or dependence begin to appear. But the manufacturer and other advocates of the drug note the cases were occurring among people with a history of substance abuse problems. (These drugs are a danger only to a small number of "addiction prone" people, they claim.) But this is no different from other adverse effects that typically first affect a body system that is already weakened or vulnerable. As time passes, more and more dependency cases emerge among people with no history of substance abuse problems. Finally, media publicity, warnings, and restrictions on prescription refills reduce the problem—but by no means eliminate it. By then the next panacea drug—with new potential problems—has appeared and is being publicized enthusiastically and uncritically.

To put all these adverse effects on human behavior into a

broader perspective, note that few if any of these cases—numbering in the hundreds of thousands—would be included in the tally of serious injuries reported in chapter 3. But they may have a more dramatic and damaging effect on people's lives than the classic adverse reactions—a perforated ulcer, a damaged liver, an allergic reaction, or a frightening episode of a runaway rapid heartbeat. We can only guess at the incidence of serious behavioral adverse reactions. However, I believe it likely that the behavioral injury toll may be as large or larger than all other adverse reactions combined, affecting millions of people every year.

CHAPTER SIX

The Threat to Cells

THE SURVIVAL OF EACH person, and the human species, depends on the delicate dance through which cells are created and destroyed. While heart, brain, and muscle cells last a lifetime, other cells are born every day. The body needs a constantly renewed supply of white blood cells to fight infection. Red blood cells wear out in a few weeks and must be discarded. The skin and hair grow continuously. The propagation of the human species is achieved through an amazing, sensitive, and frequently fallible form of cell division. The union of a single egg and sperm multiples a trillionfold to become an infant. But when the cells multiply uncontrollably in the body, the result can be cancer, our most feared killer.

Cell death is a rival to cell division in biological importance. When a cell is damaged, or when an error occurs in the complex steps of cell division, the faulty cells must be destroyed. In programmed cell death—known as apoptosis—a living cell organizes its own demise, shriveling up into a neat package that can be readily consumed by patrolling garbage scavengers—the phagocytes. Programmed cell death is also critical to the development of a human embryo—eliminating unwanted features such as gills, flippers, and webbed hands and feet. Through apoptosis a human infant is sculpted out of the cruder block of living raw material created by cell division.

Many prescription drugs can disrupt the sensitive business of cell birth and cell death, sometimes with lethal consequences. They are capable of compromising the most important cell division functions, causing cancer, birth defects, and life-threatening blood disorders. Nearly half of all drugs tested cause cancer in animals. More than 90 percent of drugs are potentially hazardous to pregnant women. One out of eight drugs can damage the bone marrow—the critical source of new red and white blood cells. At the very frontiers of science, researchers now suspect that some drugs may block apoptosis, or programmed cell death. This could provide a cancer risk that might not be detected in routine animal studies. These are the key findings that will be explored in this chapter. However, it is also important to keep these frightening facts in perspective, because threats to cell division are among the most elusive hazard of drugs. In some cases, the adverse effects are very rare, but often lethal in the cases that are reported. In other cases, the evidence of danger is indirect, from animal or laboratory testing. The applicability of the findings to humans is not certain. The process of cell division is so vital to life, and the number of drugs potentially implicated so large, it is a tragedy that so little is known. A look at one of the most important discoveries in history about drugs and cell division reveals much about how such risks are first identified.

William McBride, an obstetrician in Sydney, Australia, became curious about unusual birth defects in three babies he had delivered in six weeks' time.[1] For an obstetrician, it is not unusual to see congenital defects—they occur in 1.5 to 2 percent of newborn babies. But each of these babies had an unusual defect McBride had never seen before. Their arms had never developed a radius, the large bone in the forearm. As a result, the babies' hands were attached to the stumps of elbows. The newborns also had malformed digestive tracts, a problem that led to their deaths despite attempts at surgical repair. This particular birth defect was listed in the medical textbooks. But it was so rare that many texts used a famous painting by Salvador Dali of such a child instead of a photograph. McBride saw three cases in a few weeks' time. As he pored over the medical records of the three cases, he could find only one factor in common. The only drug that the mothers had taken during pregnancy was a sedative called Distaval. It was June of 1961.

McBride described the cases in a letter to the famed British medical journal, the *Lancet*, and to the Australian distributor of the drug. He further sought confirmation by conducting a crude animal study. He fed large but unmeasured amounts of crushed Distaval tablets to pregnant mice and guinea pigs. No abnormalities in offspring were noted. Furthermore, in the next three months, another twenty-six mothers who had taken Distaval during pregnancy gave birth at McBride's hospital. All the infants were normal. As a final blow to his suspicions about Distaval, the *Lancet* returned his letter about the three cases with a polite letter of rejection. At the time, Distaval was in widespread use around the world, a best-seller in Germany, popular in Britain, Italy, and South America. The FDA was being pressured to approve it in the United States, and more than 2 million tablets had been distributed free to doctors, who were encouraged to use it and report their experiences. The drug was called Distaval in Australia and Britain, Contergan in Germany, and Kevadon in the United States. However, the world will not forget its chemical name: thalidomide.

McBride's report ultimately reached the German company that had invented the drug and licensed it for international use. Until then, similar reports in Germany had been dismissed as the result of some bizarre virus. The postwar world was experiencing its first major drug catastrophe. Although many more would follow, none would leave as haunting an image in the public mind as the horrifying pictures of babies born without arms or legs, or with flippers, or with a few fingers attached to an elbow. In all, about 8,000 malformed infants survived thalidomide; thousands more perished. In the United States, just 17 cases occurred because of the drug samples and from women who obtained the drug abroad.[2]

More than thirty years after the thalidomide tragedy, every new prescription drug today is in some fashion assessed for its dangers to pregnant women. The results of this testing should be of serious concern. Of the 3,200 approved prescription drugs, only 6 are reported safe for pregnant women on the basis of evidence from human studies.[3] Five are thyroid hormone replacement drugs and the sixth is a form of folic acid—an important vitamin that helps prevent birth defects. Another 205 drugs produced no birth defects or other abnormalities when tested in rabbits and rats.[4] The manufacturers of these drugs note that these animal test results do not assure that they won't harm the human fetus. However, since it is unthinkable to recruit pregnant women to test the safety of these drugs, we are forced to make an assumption. Therefore, we can be comforted by the absence of evidence of harm in animal testing. However, it is not so comforting to realize that animal or human evidence provides a clean bill of health to only 211 of 3,200 approved drugs.

A large majority of drugs in widespread use either failed the animal reproduction tests or are so old they were never tested.

For safety's sake, the older drugs are assumed to have failed, absent evidence to the contrary. However, the animal results seldom translate directly to effects in humans. For example, even thalidomide did not produce the distinctive abnormal limbs in mice. However, it did show clear toxicity, with 40 to 50 percent of the fetuses being reabsorbed, and 10 to 15 percent born with defects such as cleft palate, cataracts, and deformed tails.[5] In rats, thalidomide did not cause birth defects, but many of the fetuses were reabsorbed. The animal study results of widely used drugs constitute a bizarre catalog of what can go wrong. The epilepsy drug Tegretol causes kinked ribs in rats. The painkiller Indocin causes development of abnormal blood vessels supplying the lungs. The antibiotic Floxin causes fetal deaths and "skeletal variations," while the cholesterol-lowering drug Mevacor causes skeletal malformations. The antidepressant Paxil had no mutating effect on the offspring but impaired the fertility of the parents; it caused irregular growths in sexual organs and atrophy of the testicles in male rats. Among the females, giving Paxil resulted in fewer pregnancies, more fetal losses, and "decreases viability" of the newborns.[6]

The above findings are from animal studies. For 1 out of 7 approved drugs, the evidence of birth defects comes from human experience. In many cases, however, the dire manufacturers' warnings concern drugs that a pregnant woman, or a woman who might become pregnant, would typically avoid. So birth defect warnings are made for male sex hormones, for contraceptive drugs, for the highly toxic anticancer drugs. However, other drugs that may cause birth defects in humans are much more commonly used: tranquilizers such as Xanax and Halcion; the cholesterol-lowering drug Pravachol, the smoking-cessation aids Nicoderm and Nicotrol; drugs for epilepsy such as Depakote. Here is how 1,152 drugs—now formally FDA-rated for safety—stack up:

PREGNANCY HAZARD[7]	NUMBER OF DRUGS
Safe—human evidence	6
Safe—animal studies	206
Potentially dangerous—animal evidence*	774
Dangerous—human evidence	166

*Includes rated drugs for which no animal testing was reported.

Drugs that cause birth defects frequently are linked to other cell division problems that may be harder to identify. It is still another proof that the biologically potent molecules of modern drugs affect more control switches than their designers imagined or intended. The birth of a deformed baby is the most tragic, arresting evidence of cell division error. However, the next major cell division disorder causes many more cases of death and serious injury but is much more difficult to identify in specific cases.

When cells multiply uncontrollably, the result can be cancer. It is a disease of vast extent, with more that 1 million new cases each year and about 500,000 deaths, about 1 out of every 4 deaths that occur for any reason.[8] Despite the intense medical scrutiny given to every detected cancer, the cause of a specific case usually remains a complete mystery. For example, a metastasizing breast or prostate cancer leave few clues behind about what caused it. The notable exception is that cigarette smoking is blamed for 70 to 90 percent of the 170,000 lung cancer cases identified each year, and evidence of lung damage from smoking is clinically evident in more than half of diagnosed cases.[9] However, the more that is learned about cancer, the harder it becomes to identify any single casual agent. A malignant cancer is the end product of a process that may have begun ten or twenty years earlier with damage to the DNA in only a few cells, an event called initiation.[10] Other chemical agents serve as promoters, encouraging the growth of abnormal cells that may divide slowly but still provide no mortal threat. The effects of cancer promoters are believed reversible if exposure is halted before the final phase—when cells multiply rapidly and uncontrollably. Finally, chemicals—including drugs—may disrupt the body's own mechanisms that destroy aberrant cells before they become malignant cancers.[11]

Despite the complexity of cancer causation, prescription drugs ought to be ranked second only to cigarette smoking as a cancer hazard. While certain industrial chemicals are more potent carcinogens than any drug, there are few chemical agents to which so many people are exposed at relatively high doses for great lengths of time. The evidence implicating drugs is based on both the results of animal studies and observations in humans. A frequently cited overview of cancer risks blames drugs and radiation treatment for 2,500 to 15,000 cancer deaths each year.[12] But this study contains so many estimates and crude approximations that the total could easily be five or ten times higher. The most systematic scientific evidence of cancer hazards comes from animal studies.

Among those tested, the latest survey shows that 42 percent of approved prescription drugs caused cancer in at least one species of animals.[13] Among those drugs showing cancer activity in animals, 10 percent directly damaged cell DNA and caused cancer causation outside human studies. Two-thirds of the animal carcinogens produced tumors in every animal species in which they were tested—another strong indication of cancer risk. The remainder caused tumors in one species—for example, mice—but showed no activity in another—for example, rats. These were the findings of a 1994 survey of 242 newer drugs—every one with animal test results reported on the drug's disclosure label. Another 27 drugs contain cancer warnings based on risks to humans, rather than animals.[14]

Overall, this evidence suggests about half of prescription drugs are potentially carcinogenic.[15]

What kind of risks do animal carcinogens pose to humans? A leading toxicology textbook says, "All known chemical carcinogens in humans, with the possible exception of arsenic, are carcinogenic in some species but not in all laboratory animals."[16] In other words, when researchers studied a clear human carcinogen, it also proved to cause cancer in animals. But the results were not consistent and predictable. A human carcinogen might not cause the same kind of cancer in animals that it did in humans. For example, a synthetic sex hormone caused cancer in the reproductive organs of women, but caused cancers of the adrenal and pituitary glands in rats.[17] Starting with a proven human carcinogen, researchers may not see cancers in every species tested. The abnormal growths seen in testing might be classified as "benign."[18] The cancers might occur in animal organs or biological structures that don't exist in humans. But in every case except arsenic, a human carcinogen was also an animal carcinogen. However, a controversy still rages today about the opposite question. Do animal carcinogens reliably predict danger to humans? A notable case is dioxin—one of the most virulent carcinogens ever found in animals.[19] Dioxin is so toxic that it caused cancer in mice in trace amounts so tiny it could barely be detected with the most advanced equipment. Nevertheless, similar effects have not been identified in humans accidentally exposed to high concentrations of dioxin.[20] While dioxin may—or may not—ultimately prove an exception to the animal-human link for cancer testing, it would be foolish to abandon the entire body of evidence because of a single possible exception. But that is the case advanced by some who want to relax controls on pesticides and environmental contaminants, arguing that evidence of cancer must come from human studies.

Unrealistically high doses are the second objection to relying on animal studies. In standard animal toxicology tests, mice or rats are fed the maximum dose they can tolerate for their lifetime of two or three years. When studying food additives or some pesticides, this means animal doses that caused cancer could reach 380,000 times the likely human exposure.[21] With prescription drugs, however, animal cancers are often seen near the comparable human dose.[22] This is because animals can rarely tolerate unrealistically large amounts of potent prescription drugs. With pesticide testing, animals may not be able to tolerate an enormous dose, but humans would be exposed to minute trace amounts on fruits, vegetables, or other produce. However, humans typically ingest a drug continuously for many years. Thus, when prescription drugs flunk their animal cancer tests, it is often at exposures in the neighborhood of a typical human dose over time. For example, salmon calcitonin, now being promoted as a long-term treatment for osteoporosis in older women, caused cancer in both rats and mice at lower doses than the manufacturer recommended for humans.[23] The aggressively marketed new calcium channel blocker Plendil caused cancers in animals at 2.8 to 28 times the human dose in two years' time. A typical patient would take Plendil for many years, and thus would likely exceed the exposure that caused cancer in rats. The epilepsy drug Depakene produced tumors in rats and mice at less than the human dosage.[24]

Some classes of drugs evidently carried special cancer risks. The survey quoted above showed that 83 percent of cholesterol-lowering drugs caused cancer in animals; 87 percent of the cancer chemotherapy agents tested were implicated. On the other hand, only half the antibiotics and about 40 percent of the psychologically active drugs flunked animal cancer testing.

Sometimes drugs get a clean bill of health on cancer for a dangerous reason: they are too toxic for the animals even at the human dosage. For example, none of fourteen anti-inflammatory painkillers tested caused cancer in animals. However, the animal tests had to be conducted at unrealistically low doses because the drugs were so toxic to the gastrointestinal tract and kidneys—just as they are in humans.[25] For example, Orudis was so toxic to mice that they could tolerate only half the comparable human dose.[26] The animal tests for Anaprox, or naproxen, were only at 23 percent of the human dose because of the same toxicity problems.

How much exposure to a carcinogen through prescription drugs is too much? One existing standard from a leading toxicology textbook is a safety factor of 100. First, a chemical should be free of carcinogenic effects at at least 10 times the human exposure because some humans will be especially vulnerable to cancer, or to that chemical.[27] An additional safety factor of 10 is added because a weak carcinogen in animals could be more potent in humans.[28] By this standard, it would be hard to find any drug that qualified as safe. Prescription drugs are so inherently toxic that animals could tolerate few if any drugs at 100 times the expected human exposure. Even at the tolerated dose, almost half cause cancer.

At the pinnacle of the cancer risk pyramid are twenty-four chemicals—including asbestos, radon, and vinyl chloride—that are officially identified as causing cancer in humans. This list of cancer-causing chemicals is reviewed by expert panels convened by the National Toxicology Program to assess all the evidence. Few chemicals make the list. This is not so much because anyone is confident the others are safe but because the scientific evidence is lacking to declare with confidence that they cause cancer. These toxicology review panels are conservative about evidence. Among the human carcinogens thus identified, 42 percent are prescription drugs.[29] The story of one of those proven human carcinogens teaches much about modern society's ability to identify and control cancer hazards.

A young gynecologist and obstetrician named Arthur Herbst encountered a medical event almost as rare as the birth defects that provoked the curiosity of William McBride in Australia. The year was 1966 and Herbst was then a member of the Harvard University faculty at Massachusetts General Hospital in Boston. One day, he examined a fifteen-year-old girl complaining of a fairly common symptom—irregular menstrual bleeding. Upon examination, the girl was found to have clear-cell cancer of the vagina.[30] Cancer in young girls is rare under any circumstances; this particular form of cancer was itself rare at any age and practically unheard of in young women. At the famed Massachusetts General Hospital, there was no record of anyone having ever seen a similar case. Over the next three years, Herbst and his colleagues saw seven more cases, all in young women born between 1946 and 1951. Their curiosity provoked, they launched a detailed study to find some factor these young girls had in common. They checked their weight at birth, and their age when menstruation began. They asked about rare illnesses and cigarette smoking. They even scrutinized the cosmetics the young women used and asked about household pets. Nothing was found. Then they focused on the cancer victims' mothers and fathers. What was their occupation? Did they drink alcohol? Did they have any noteworthy illnesses? What kind of cosmetics did the mothers use? Did they breast-feed their daughters? No telltale clusters emerged. Finally, one of the mothers volunteered the solution to the mystery. She said that she had taken an estrogen drug called DES during pregnancy, prescribed to prevent spontaneous abortion and miscarriage. When investigators asked the other seven mothers, all but one reported taking DES.

The drug DES—or diethylstilbestrol—already had a troubled history in medicine. A synthetic form of estrogen, it became widely used in the late 1940s in pregnant women on the untested theory that it ought to reduce complications in pregnancy. In 1953, a team at the University of Chicago put DES to the classic test in a randomized, double-blind clinical trial. They found it had no benefit; a later analysis suggested it was even harmful.[31] After the study, prescription volume declined slowly, but hundreds of thousands of women still received the drug. Almost twenty years passed before Herbst and his colleagues published their findings in the *New England Journal of Medicine*, in June 1971.

The discovery was, as the accompanying editorial said, "of great scientific importance and serious social implication."[32] First, a widely used prescription drug caused cancer in humans. Also, the cancers had appeared in offspring—a population group at which no one had ever dreamed of looking for the effects of carcinogens. Finally, it was still another reminder that thalidomide was hardly the only drug capable of harming a developing human fetus. The fetus was proving remarkably vulnerable to harm from a wide range of chemicals—with drugs numbering first among them. The discovery was also of no comfort to those under the illusion that society was doing an adequate job of monitoring the cancer risks of drugs and other chemicals. Both Herbst and McBride spotted the dangerous consequences of the drug by the merest quirk of fate. By chance, the two drugs—thalidomide and DES— happened to cause a medical disorder so rare and distinctive that it provoked the curiosity of these alert physicians. But they could have never spotted an even more lethal drug that produced a much more common disorder. If the drugs had caused one of the common congenital birth defects, the cases would have been ignored as an everyday occurrence. It is likely that the capacity of drugs to cause cancer in humans is not so rare. What is unusual is an effect so distinctive it can be detected.

With a confirming study, media attention, and an FDA warning, the use of DES in pregnant women gradually declined—but did not disappear entirely.[33] DES is still on the market today. When the cancer risk was first discovered, the American Medical Association was more concerned about maintaining patient confidence than warning about the dangers of DES. "Since the risk is small, it may not be wise to stir a national alarm," noted an editorial in the association journal.[34] Although the logic is troubling, the risk of cancer was in fact small. Among roughly 3 million offspring exposed to DES between 1947 and 1975, only a few hundred cases of vaginal cancer were diagnosed and reported.[35]

While cancer in the offspring was rare, DES caused abnormal sexual organs in hundred of thousands of cases. In females, it caused irregular cell growths in the vagina, including transverse ridges, collars, hoods, cockscombs, and sulci. In males, it was associated with underdeveloped and undescended testicles, cysts in the sperm ducts, and undersized penises. In the populations reported in published medical studies, abnormalities were seen in about one-third of the female offspring, and one-quarter of the males.[36] Literally hundreds of thousands of offspring had abnormal sexual organs because of exposure to DES. This generation is today in their thirties and forties. (As the women approached thirty, the abnormal growths tended to disappear spontaneously; however, these women often developed fertility problems.) Just a few years later, a second drug was implicated in cancer, and this time the number of cancer cases would be far larger.

In the year 1975, a young Seattle medical researcher named Noel Weiss had an impressive résumé and an interest in cancer prevention. He had been awarded two different doctor's degrees—one in medicine and another in public health and epidemiology. With a fellowship at the National Center for Health Statistics, Weiss had further honed his skills in spotting new trends in health and disease. Part of Weiss's job was to help set up the Washington State reporting for a new national cancer registry then being established by the National Cancer Institute. Hardly anyone in the country was better trained and better situated to spot a new trend in cancer. Weiss soon saw something in his first Washington State data. There were almost twice as many cases of cancer of the uterus as expected. His curiosity provoked, he began to look at data from other regions that had been collected for a longer time. He became convinced that the nation was experiencing an epidemic of the most common cancer of the uterus, endometrial cancer. In just three or four years, endometrial cancer rates had about doubled.

Weiss had one suspect for the rapid rise in endometrial cancer: estrogen replacement after menopause. For more than ten years, it had been known that estrogen had a liability as well as the benefit of relieving symptoms of menopause. Providing continuous estrogen where there was no monthly cycle of menstruation caused cell growth to accumulate in the sensitive lining of the uterus. And Weiss had earlier wondered whether this cell growth might become cancerous in some cases. Drug prescriptions for estrogen had been rising rapidly, with use doubling in some regions of the United States over the preceding decade. Now, according to the new data, so was the incidence of endometrial cancer. Weiss wrote up the results, citing the biological evidence and the trends in estrogen use, and submitted a paper to the *New England Journal of Medicine*. It was politely rejected.

One year later, Weiss got a curious call from the *New England Journal*. Would Weiss care to resubmit his paper? This time they were very interested. In fact, there had been an admitted weakness in Weiss's case against estrogen. The alarming rise in endometrial cancer was real, as was the rapid increase in estrogen use. But the evidence linking the two trends, while plausible, was thin. In the intervening year, the journal had received two studies of a quite different kind. Researchers had studied groups of women who had been diagnosed with endometrial cancer. In both groups, estrogen use proved to be the largest and most important risk factor. The three papers, published together in June 1976, made a compelling case about the drug.[37] Other case control studies confirmed these results.[38] With long-term use of about five years or more, women taking Premarin and similar estrogen replacement drugs were eight times more likely to be diagnosed with endometrial cancer.

Those observing trends in cancer of the uterus warned of a cancer epidemic, with 15,000 cases of endometrial cancer linked to estrogen in the 1970-to-1975 period alone, with new cases occurring at a rate of about 7,000 every year. Such are the unsolved mysteries of cancer causation that it is extremely rare to find the cause of a major rise in cancer incidence. Cigarette smoking and lung cancer in men was the first such culprit clearly identified. The second was a prescription drug. Hershel Jick of the Boston Collaborative Drug Surveillance Program said estrogen caused "one of the largest epidemics of serious disease" ever to result from medical treatment in the United States.[39]

However, it is important to keep the risks of prescription drugs in the same measured perspective as the benefits. Even when the link to cancer is strong, the absolute risk may be quite small. As noted, among nearly 3 million women exposed to DES, only a few hundred cancer cases were reported among offspring. Weiss estimates that after five years of unopposed estrogen therapy a woman has a 1-in-200 annual chance of endometrial cancer; after ten years the risk is 1 in 100 per year.[40] Some might consider this a small risk. However, it is one of the highest in the medical literature. For example the annual incidence of lung cancer in asbestos workers who had smoked was 1 in 250.[41] The risk in men with a history of heavy smoking is similar. (It should be noted, however, that the five-year survival rate for endometrial cancer is much higher than that for lung cancer—83 percent versus 13 percent.[42] Among cases specifically attributed to estrogen therapy, the survival rate could be even better.)

The avalanche of cancer studies and an FDA warning led to a steady decline in prescriptions for estrogen—from about 29 million prescriptions in 1975 to 15 million prescriptions in 1980.[43] In the mid-1980s, estrogen's fortunes were revived in part by evidence that the high risk of endometrial cancer might be eliminated by adding a second major sex hormone—progesterone—to hormone replacement therapy. This made biological sense. Unopposed, continuous estrogen was stimulating overgrowth of the cells lining the wall of the uterus. In some women, some of these cells developed into precancerous polyps and cysts. Some of these became outright cancers, proliferating malignantly. Adding progesterone to the monthly cycle eliminated the early part of the problem—the accumulation of cell growth in the lining of the uterus. Additional studies of women taking both hormones did not detect the elevated cancer risk seen in women taking unopposed estrogen for five years or more.[44] Unfortunately, this seemingly clean bill of health is not nearly as well documented as the original hazard. It is part of the age-old tendency to be much less critical about claims for benefits than about risks.

The female sex hormones are powerful cell growth stimulators and their use in prescription drugs can result in cancer. This was true of estrogen given to pregnant women, and of estrogen given to women after menopause. Liver cancer is a documented risk of using estrogen-based contraceptives.[45] It would not be surprising if larger studies confirm several existing reports that estrogen also increases the risk of breast cancer.[45]

It is amazing that all these questions about estrogen did not lead to clinical trials to measure the net risks and benefits of long-term therapy. As we shall see later, the long-term effects of drugs both good and bad are rarely determined, no matter how many millions of people may be at risk. This leaves women today with guesswork about the overall health risks. On the positive side is evidence that estrogen slows the process of osteoporosis and helps to prevent hip and arm fractures late in life. It also may reduce substantially the risk of heart disease. Those directly concerned about a personal decision on estrogen should consult the summary of the evidence and uncertainties published by the American College of Physicians.[47]

For the rest of us, the overall cancer risks of drugs remain poorly defined, widely ignored, and the subject of little if any clinical research. But toxicologists warn that even statistically small cancer risks can produce large numbers of cases. "Consider that a 0.5 percent increase in cancer incidence in the United States would result in over 1 million additional cancer deaths each year—clearly an unacceptably high risk," notes a major toxicology textbook.[48] Our society could be more relaxed about these poorly understood risks if more progress were being made in reducing cancer deaths. While death rates from heart disease, stroke, and most other disorders have declined dramatically over the last twenty-five years, cancer death rates crept slowly upward until 1990, then leveled off. But all the billions spent for cancer detection and treatment have not produced the expected progress.[49] No one knows the reason for these disappointing results. In the cancer establishment, little has been said or written about this major failure of the war on cancer to make significant overall gains.

The other major threat to cell division gets possibly even less attention than the cancer risks of prescription drugs. For reasons that are not understood, and in relatively rare cases, prescription drugs are capable of destroying or severely impairing the bone marrow, which produces a life-sustaining supply of red and white blood cells.

The first signs of bone marrow damage are subtle and insidious. The final stages of complete bone marrow failure cause a ghastly death. The first identifiable symptom can be a nagging sore throat that won't go away, or a cut that will not heal. In the presence of these symptoms, a blood test may document a mysterious shortage of the most common white blood cell generated by the bone marrow, the granulocyte. This problem has the medical name of agranulocytosis. Because these cells die in a matter of hours, they are the first sign of damage to the bone marrow. The next medical problems arise from lack of platelets, which live six or seven days. Without platelets to form blood clots, the patient begins to bleed from any vulnerable spot. Even mild pressure on an area of exposed skin can lead to a large black bruise. Finally, the victim begins to suffer from lack of the longest-lived blood cells—the red blood cells. The initial effect is anemia, shortness of breath, and a ghostly pallor. Unless the bone marrow can somehow be restored, the result is a shattered body riddled with infection, blackened by internal bleeding and bruises and starved for oxygen. About 30 percent of the cases are fatal. Although little known to the public, this condition, called aplastic anemia, is among doctors one of the most feared complication of prescription drugs.

At least 133 drugs contain disclosure warnings that they may be capable of causing aplastic anemia. The list includes such widely used drugs as Zantac, Prozac, Motrin, and Floxin, the wide-spectrum antibiotic. Although one of the most serious and feared of all adverse effects of drugs, it is apparently quite rare, except in drugs used to treat cancer. In one of the best studied of all cases, the antibiotic chloramphenicol caused aplastic anemia in about 1 in 30,000 cases.[50] In the case of Prozac, aplastic anemia is so rare that the manufacturer acknowledges that a few such cases have been reported among the millions who have taken the drug, and a causal relationship not firmly established.

Even when a new drug that causes aplastic anemia is positively identified, it often leaves doctor and patient little wiser. In 1993, Carter-Wallace began marketing Felbatol, a new drug for epilepsy and other seizures. No special problems were noted in the initial drug testing, which was limited to a few hundred patients. However, in the first year the FDA identified ten cases of aplastic anemia, including two fatalities. A warning was mailed to doctors, but no one could say how serious the danger might be. Other than to say that Felbatol increased the risk of aplastic anemia by a hundredfold, the FDA could not tell how frequently the cases occurred, at what dose, or whether the risk continued among epilepsy patients successfully treated with Felbatol without observable adverse effects.[51]

Prescription drugs are the only known cause of the milder and more common bone marrow problem, granulocytosis. In a blood test, granulocytes are the most frequently found white blood cells. In this disorder, the granulocytes disappear or their number is drastically reduced. This disease was discovered in 1933 when two Milwaukee researchers finally identified the cause of a puzzling epidemic that was then occurring. It was being caused by a popular painkiller of the time, amidopyrine.[52] Before the discovery of antibiotics, agranulocytosis frequently led to death from infections that could not be controlled by a compromised immune system. Today, antibiotics usually can hold infection at bay while the offending drug is removed and the white blood cells regenerate.

Are the harmful effects of drugs on bone marrow too rare to worry about? The FDA studied computerized death certificates for one year and found 4,490 deaths.[53] That is more deaths than occur from all fires, or boating accidents, and about the same as the total for all workplace injuries. The investigators, however, were stymied by the same reporting failure for drug-related deaths noted earlier. In fact, they could identify a drug in only 2 percent of the certificates. Radiation and certain industrial chemicals such as benzene can also cause aplastic anemia, so prescription drugs can't be blamed in every case. Bone marrow damage is still another of the risks of prescription drugs that are so poorly researched that an accurate assessment of the peril is simply not possible.

Some drugs are so toxic that they have damaging effects on all the major cell division functions—not just one. The acne medication Accutane is the classic example.

In its capacity to cause birth defects, Accutane has few equals, including thalidomide. The manufacturer warns the risk of a deformed infant is "extremely high."[54] It has caused babies to be born with grossly enlarged skulls, with undersized or absent ears, and mishappen eyes, cleft palates, and distorted faces. Other infants had malfunctioning thyroid or thymus glands. Even when the infants look normal, the manufacturer warns, they may have an IQ below 85.

While Accutane is not officially reported to cause the two major blood disorders—aplastic anemia or agranulocytosis—there is evidence it may damage the bone marrow. From 10 to 25 percent of Accutane patients show reduced numbers of red and white blood cells, but abnormally large numbers of the clot-causing platelets. If that were not enough of a warning sign, the manufacturer acknowledges reports of many symptoms that could indicate a bone marrow disorder, including bruising, abnormal menstruation, anemia, respiratory infection, and bleeding gums.

The findings for cancer were no more reassuring. Accutane caused cancer in rats at four times the human dose (measured by the lenient standard of weight) in eighteen months' time.[55] It showed "weakly positive" effects on one cell mutation test— suggesting an effect on cell DNA. Many of those laboratory animals that didn't get cancer developed other severe health problems. Among the most dangerous were fibrous growths and inflammation of the heart, calcification of the heart and blood vessels, and clouded corneas of the eyes. When researchers checked to see if the same effects on the eyes could be found in humans, the danger was confirmed. Five of seventy-two patients examined had "corneal opacities."[56]

Of all the adverse effects of drugs, the effects on cell division are likely the most underestimated hazard. Investigation is more difficult because the effects, while very serious, are typically quite rare and do not appear in the routine testing of new drugs. But because the exposure of the public is so large, it is likely that bone marrow injury by drugs results in thousands of deaths and tens of thousands of hospitalizations every year. That so little is known about these risks should not be confused with their potential importance. Unknown and poorly measured hazards often provide greater dangers than more familiar fears.

PART TWO

A FLAWED SYSTEM

CHAPTER SEVEN

The System

As THIS BOOK BEGAN, Amy Kaufman lay dead of cardiac arrest after taking one extra tablet of an antihistamine called Hismanal. In a later chapter, a depressed young mother normally given to fits of crying alone took Prozac and was hospitalized for mania after attacking three policemen. A San Francisco psychiatrist named John Mudd got off his bicycle and collapsed in cardiac arrest after taking Tambocor for a mild irregular heartbeat. A case of free samples of addictive cough syrup helped ruin the medical career of Christopher Iliades, the Boston doctor. These stories dramatize the dangers of drugs. To explore how such risks may be controlled requires a change in focus. The next chapters will examine how drugs are tested, approved, and prescribed. The path to greater safety lies not in the drugs themselves but in strengthening the system that provides them. Seen as a system, problems may emerge in any of these links in the safety chain:

- Before being marketed to millions of people, the drugs must be adequately tested. However, inadequate drug testing has resulted in thousands of deaths, frequent restrictions, and a flood of warnings about new and severe adverse effects.

- Once approved, the safety of the drugs must be closely monitored. The United States government has more federal employees at the Naval Academy Laundry (107) than assigned to monitor the safety of approved drugs (54).[1] Because this tiny FDA staff has no reliable count of deaths or serious injuries, no one knows whether the national is gaining or losing ground on drug safety.

- The manufactured drug must be free of contamination. However, drug recalls occur every week, and some drug companies have severe quality control problems.

- The doctor must prescribe the right drug, in the right dose, for a correctly diagnosed disorder. Inappropriate drugs were prescribed for 1 out of 5 elderly patients, one survey showed. In another study, 60 percent of the patients went home with a drug that wouldn't benefit them.

- The pharmacist must dispense the prescription accurately, and check for drug interactions and other errors. But in one report, a third of the pharmacies checked filled two prescriptions with a potentially lethal interaction.

- Consumers should be alert to the risks of the drugs and should take them as prescribed. However, the most dire warnings issued by manufacturers seldom reach consumers. Also, approximately one-half of drug doses are not taken as prescribed, sometimes with serious medical consequences.

———

As this brief summary shows, a problem in any single link in the safety chain can jeopardize lives needlessly. A closer examination reveals some strengths and many glaring weaknesses in the individual components of the system.

Society's primary response to the dangers of prescription drugs has been to demand extensive testing before their widespread use. This is the point at which the system's standards are most rigorous, requiring elaborate laboratory studies, scientific testing in hundreds of humans and several species of animals. About 9 out of 10 drugs that are promising enough to enter human testing do not enter the marketplace, even though millions may have been spent in basic research and preclinical studies.[2] Requiring rigorous testing before approval is sound public policy on several grounds. History shows that most—but not all—drug catastrophes were a result of inadequate initial testing. More rigorous scientific scrutiny at the start would have prevented tens of thousands of deaths and serious injuries. Also, many adverse effects of drugs simply cannot be detected without the expensive, systematic scientific study that is typically undertaken only to win approval. Without such studies, people may be injured perpetually. For example, one study of drugs withdrawn for safety reasons showed that they had remained on the market for an average of twenty-eight years.[3] Earlier chapters have shown the propensity of doctors and patients alike to embrace uncritically new treatments that scientific study reveals as harmful or ineffective. Finally, even drugs with important new benefits may be harmful if given in the wrong dose, or to the wrong patients. Thousands of people were unnecessarily injured by the valuable AIDS drug AZT because health authorities rushed to use it in patient populations in which it had not been tested. However, these entry barriers extract a price that has been much advertised. It means delays of several years while a new treatment is tested. It means that some promising chemicals may never be tested because no company or government is willing to invest the large sums required.

Initial drug testing in humans and animals usually takes four to five years and costs about $1.5 million.[4] The West European democracies, Canada, the United States, and Japan operate roughly similar systems. The drug companies are entirely responsible for conducting the actual testing. The regulating agencies evaluate the results. The FDA in the United States is known for its detailed requirements and careful scrutiny. FDA staff members check on the caged rats in animal testing centers. Inspectors call on the research physicians doing the human testing. They check their credentials and audit the patient records—sometimes detecting fraud.[5] Practically all the test results—often tens of thousands of pages—are submitted to the FDA for review. (Some European countries accept summaries.) At the FDA, the reviewing team includes a medical doctor to evaluate the results in humans, a chemist to assess the structure and stability of the molecule itself, and a toxicologist to review the animal studies. It takes four to five months for the evaluators just to read through and absorb this enormous mass of data. The team's evaluation report is reviewed at three higher levels before final approval or disapproval. It currently takes the FDA an average of sixteen months to evaluate and approve a new drug; review times at the major European drug agencies are similar.[6] For breakthrough drugs, the FDA has acted within a few months under crash programs. Overall, it typically takes about ten years for a new drug to reach the public—counting all the time needed to identify a promising new molecule, complete the animal and human testing, and obtain government approval. In a crash program, the newest generation of AIDS drugs made the journey in approximately half that time.

In order to hurry a new drug to market, the FDA approves drugs for marketing while important safety questions remain unanswered. For example, the FDA knew that a heart drug called Norpace might be dangerous in patients with heart failure. But it didn't want to delay approval while the additional study was completed. Hundreds died because Norpace proved more harmful in these patients than suspected.[7] The FDA approved a new painkiller called Ultram that had chemical similarities to narcotics. So as not to delay approval, the FDA allowed the company to study Ultram's addictive properties while marketing it as a nonaddictive painkiller. In the first months after its approval, the FDA received numerous reports suggesting a danger of addiction. A special warning letter was sent to doctors.[8] Rather than being the strict, overcautious organization its critics claim, the FDA has repeatedly compromised on safety questions to help drug companies get their new product on the market more quickly or meet other public pressures. While the FDA can be strict and inflexible in insisting on scientific proof that a drug has a medical effect, it can sometimes be flexible on questions of safety.

Some important questions are rarely answered about drugs, either before approval or afterward. For example, new drugs are not tested separately in the elderly—a group that often responds differently to drugs. The typical human trials are too small and too short to detect some of the most serious but rare side effects—such as cancer or damage to the bone marrow. And the FDA almost never requires long-term testing for drugs intended for long-term use. Thus, a new drug for depression called Effexor was tested for efficiency for only six weeks.[9] When the best-selling cholesterol drug Mevacor was approved for lifetime therapy, fewer than two hundred people had taken it for as long as two years.[10] Thus, initial drug testing is essential but incomplete. The only systematic study in the scientific literature found that 51 percent of drugs approved over a decade's time had important risks not detectable in initial testing.[11]

This deliberate gamble with the safety of the public requires an excellent system to monitor the safety of drugs once they enter the marketplace. For example, in airline safety the FAA not only must evaluate the safety of new aircraft designs entering service, it assigns 4,000 inspectors to monitor the daily operations of 81 commercial air carriers. However, when we look at the safety monitoring of approved drugs, what actually exists can only be described as pitiful. To monitor the safety of 3,200 approved drugs taken daily by millions of people, the FDA has a staff of just 54. By comparison, to evaluate an average of 25 new drugs a year, the FDA has 1,500 chemists, doctors, toxicologists, and statistical experts.[12] Overall, only about 4 percent of the FDA budget for drug evaluation goes to monitor the safety of existing drugs, a paltry total of less than $6 million.[13] The FDA has only one Ph.D. epidemiologist and five medical doctors assigned to this task.

At the FDA, the Division of Pharmacovigilance and Epidemiology is responsible for monitoring the safety of approved drugs. To monitor the deaths and serious injuries caused by approved prescription drugs, it relies on voluntary reports. It makes no more sense to monitor the dangers of drugs with spontaneous anecdotal reports than to measure the benefits of drugs by asking doctors to volunteer stories of miraculous recoveries. To illustrate just how poorly this system operates, consider these results from an FDA-funded survey. Researchers asked every practicing doctor in the state of Rhode Island how many adverse drug reactions they remembered seeing in the past year. While relying on the memory of a physician who sees thousands of patients may not be the most accurate approach, it is unlikely to result in exaggeration. Three-quarters of the doctors in the state responded—a total of 1,035 physicians. Overall, they recalled seeing a total of 26,000 adverse reactions, including 8,000 cases so serious they resulted in hospitalization or death. In that same period, the FDA got only 11 voluntary reports directly from Rhode Island doctors, and only 55 from all sources combined in Rhode Island. How good is a system in which the doctors report only 11 of 26,000 drug injuries? We can only guess what the total would be in a study that relied on medical records or a survey of patients instead of the fallible memory of busy doctors.

So what does the FDA system reveal about deaths and injuries from adverse reactions to drugs? In 1995, the FDA received reports of 110,885 adverse reactions to drugs, including 78,837 from health professionals in the United States.[14] A majority of these reports were initially sent to drug companies, which by law must forward them to the FDA. If less than 1 percent of all adverse reactions are reported—as the Rhode Island study suggests—then something like 10 million people were injured by drugs in one year, including at least 1.6 million severely, and 300,000 killed. But the truth is this defective system can't provide that information. The real total could be lower or higher. From 1992 to 1994, the number of adverse reaction reports rose by 17 percent. Does that mean an epidemic of drug injuries? If the number of auto accidents rose by that amount, it would cause national alarm and immediate action. Or were doctors and pharmacists just being more conscientious about volunteering information about drug injuries and death? That can't be determined. This is the definition of a system fatally flawed by design. In 1996, I asked the then director of the division, Vincent Guinee, whether prescription drugs were getting safer or more dangerous in recent years. He had to answer that he didn't know. Because the system is flying blind, no one can tell how serious the problem is, or whether the situation is improving or getting worse.

Any system that takes in thousands of detailed reports every year often does reveal valuable information. It can detect new adverse effects that are too rare to observe in initial testing and distinctive enough to provoke the curiosity of an alert physician. Through this system, the FDA quickly realized in 1992, that the new antibiotic Omniflox was severely injuring patients, destroying red blood cells, dangerously lowering blood sugar, causing kidney failure, liver damage, and bleeding.[15] However, a voluntary reporting system can detect these side effects only when they are unusual or distinctive. In an adult who is healthy except for pneumonia, damage to an entirely different organ such as the liver is likely to attract a doctor's attention as possibly an adverse drug effect. However, if the adverse reaction is a very common medical problem, or similar to the effects of the disease, the voluntary reporting will fail. In most cases, the problem will be blamed on the patient's medical condition instead of the drug. For example, the cardiac drug Manoplax hastened the deaths of some patients with heart failure.[16] But the problem was invisible to the prescribing physicians because they expected the deaths of some of their heart failure patients. If the observing physicians noticed anything, it was that the drug made the symptoms of heart failure better for a short time. Only a controlled trial comparing treated to untreated patients was able to demonstrate Manoplax's capacity to create mortality. Enkaid, a drug for heart rhythm disturbances, caused cardiac arrest—but the doctors expected such events in patients with heart trouble and rarely suspected the drug.[17] Only a clinical trial uncovered the danger. Adverse reaction report systems cannot detect such adverse effects.

In addition to leaving society blind about how much damage drugs are doing, this flawed monitoring system has a more insidious and sinister defect. It leads to an illusion of safety, suggesting that the injuries reported are uncommon, and therefore, that a particular drug and the whole system is relatively sound. In 1995, reports of 3,128 suspected drug-related deaths reached the FDA—a substantial but not immediately alarming total. As noted earlier, the real total is probably much closer to 100,000 deaths a year—a number so large that drug safety ought to be an important public concern. The problem is even more insidious when a few reports accumulate about a particular drug. FDA and drug company doctors analyze the cases in depth and conclude the effect is probably real but very rare. After all, they only had a few reports! A warning is added to the drug disclosure label and everybody forgets about the problem. A study in France illustrated how easily this approach leads to drastic underestimation of drug dangers.

Cipro, Floxin, and Noroxin are a class of broad-spectrum antibiotics called fluroquinolones. In studies in dogs, these drugs caused damage to the cartilage in weight-bearing joints. It was a logical question whether patients would report rheumatismlike knee joint or muscle pains after taking these drugs. The disclosure label for Noroxin notes only that arthritis and joint pain "have been reported."[18] Based on voluntary reporting—similar to the U.S. system—the incident in France seemed extremely rare—1 in 100,000 patients. Then the French health authorities began asking doctors who called on other matters whether they had seen adverse effects. With active questioning of a few doctors—rather than spontaneous reporting—the incident immediately grew eighteenfold. Finally, in one French region, authorities canvassed every one of the doctors who had prescribed these antibiotics over a three-month period. This time, the incidence of joint pain grew to 347 cases for every 100,000 patients. Had they questioned patients instead of their doctors, it is likely more cases would have been discovered—possibly two or three times as many. In this case, the spontaneous reporting system was capturing only two-tenths of 1 percent of the events found with an active search. It is a bad system indeed that not only misses most adverse events but also produces misleading illusions of safety. The next link in the safety chain is usually stronger.

When a consumer removes a capsule from a medicine bottle, he or she assumes the drug is at full strength and free of contamination. When a woman opens a new package of the contraceptive Loestrin and takes a pill to begin a new monthly cycle, she normally expects the active drug. Parke-Davis, however, made 1.7 million dispensers with seven placebos put in the top row—instead of the bottom row for the end of the monthly menstrual cycle. When consumers open packages of Parke-Davis's Benadryl Elixir, an antihistamine, they do not expect to find glass fragments in the liquid, as occurred in 344,700 bottles. Eli Lilly made a liquid form of Prozac that leaked out of the bottles. Warner-Lambert had particular problems with Dilantin, an important epilepsy drug that prevents seizures, recalling five different batches of the drug in 1995. In fact, drug recalls are very common, with 251 recorded in 1995, a typical year. Fortunately, only one or two recalls every year involve immediately life-threatening dangers. In a more typical recall, the pills will become discolored because the wrong stopper was put into the bottle, or the pill will not dissolve as specified and therefore might not deliver a full-strength dose.

To insure product quality, the FDA deploys the equivalent of seventy-three inspectors in field offices who conduct unannounced inspections of more than two thousand pharmaceutical plants, visiting each about once every two years.[19] As in most industry safety inspection programs, the focus is on the paperwork. The company has to describe the exact process by which it manufactures the medicine. It has to maintain records of each batch of medicine and record any testing for purity and other factors. A company can't make even small changes in manufacturing without notice to the FDA.

Based on the number and kinds of violations discovered, the nation is wise to maintain a careful watch on the manufacturing process. In recent years, two of the major drug manufacturers have been taken to court over impure drugs. In 1989, federal inspectors uncovered so many deficiencies in one of Eli Lilly's major plants in Indianapolis that the company shut it down immediately. Shipments of ten different products were recalled. The FDA took Eli Lilly to court and required improvements that were made under court supervision.[20] Even worse manufacturing problems were found at Warner-Lambert and its Parke-Davis subsidiary. The number of Warner-Lambert drug recalls dwarfs that of any other pharmaceutical company. In 1992 and 1993, it had to recall fourteen different drugs, with some drugs undergoing repeated recalls. In 1993, the FDA took Warner-Lambert to court and got an order shutting down all the company's plants except for the manufacture of fourteen essential drugs. In 1995, the company was fined $10 million for withholding information about manufacturing problems. The company's stock price was not affected. It was a classic case of the recurring collision between safety and profitability. Despite years of manufacturing problems, Warner-Lambert kept its profit margins growing—from $485 million in 1990 to $694 million in 1994.[21] But to show what is at stake, Warner-Lambert's president, Lodewijk de Vink, told a trade publication that it would cost the company $1 billion to make the manufacturing improvements that the FDA was demanding under court order.[22]

After bottles of an approved drug leave the pharmaceutical manufacturing plant, the heavy hand of federal regulation abruptly disappears. The nation's 525,000 practicing physicians will now choose a particular drug for a specific patient from among the 3,200 approved drugs. Over the independence prescribing practices of physicians, there is an utter minimum of outside safety monitoring, guidance, or interference of any kind. The Drug Enforcement Administration and state medical agencies monitor prescribing practices to detect outright drug trafficking or more subtle evidence of addiction by physicians and other health professionals. However, the FDA is often emphatic that it does not regulate the practice of medicine. It tells drug companies what to do but leave the nation's doctors largely alone.

In the doctor's office, the entire system will succeed or fail. The millions of dollars of testing can be seen as an effort to provide doctors with adequate instructions for a drug's use— and accurate scientific information about its likely effects. It is the alert doctor who will spot the signs of addiction to tranquilizers and a sloppy one who will unquestioningly agree to refills at gradually increasing doses. The doctor can choose between the cheapest generic and the newest drug. The doctor can wade through a mountain of scientific literature to assess drugs carefully, or use the easy-to-read sales brochures and drug samples left by drug company sales force. The doctor can patiently explain the benefits of a drug and review the most likely adverse effects, or hand out a prescription with a minimum of comment. Doctors can be eager prescribers offering tranquilizers, sleep aids, antidepressants, cholesterol and blood pressure drugs at the first indication of a problem. Or they can be conservative, urging patients to focus on diet and nondrug alternatives before resorting to drugs. It is here that serious mistakes can be made even with drugs that are valuable and thoroughly tested. Some people believe that doctors should have very wide latitude in prescribing drugs—everything from herbal remedies to experimental gene therapy. On the other hand, others might suggest doctors should work in a tightly monitored, disciplined system as do airline pilots, whose every cockpit comment and control change is recorded in case of an accident. The following evidence shows that whatever your view, much more study is needed about how to help doctors do a better job selecting and prescribing drugs.

A group of researchers at Harvard Medical School started with a list of twenty drugs that a panel of experts had identified as too dangerous to use in elderly patients.[23] Then they examined which drugs were being prescribed for a nationwide sample of 6,171 patients over age sixty-five. They found 23 percent were receiving these inappropriate, potentially dangerous drugs. An editorial in *JAMA*, journal of the American Medical Association, described this study as merely "the tip of the iceberg."[24] Then another research team in California repeated the study, focusing on a different group of elderly patients. They found 14 percent receiving these twenty inappropriate drugs.[25] A concerned U.S. Congress noted these troubling findings and asked the federal General Accounting Office to investigate independently. The GAO, using Medicare survey data, found 17 percent of the elderly were receiving inappropriate drugs.[26]

Consider what this tells us about the system. Two groups of independent researchers showed that roughly 1 out of 5 of the elderly are being needlessly endangered because their doctors prescribed drugs that were inappropriate. These findings were not buried or concealed; on the contrary, they were published in two major peer-reviewed journals—the *Archives of Internal Medicine*, and *JAMA*. The problem attracted the attention of a concerned U.S. Congress, which requested an independent investigation that confirmed the facts a third time. Thus, we can be reasonably confident the findings are genuine and free of major scientific controversy, and that the information was available to major medical organizations, the U.S. Congress, and the FDA. So what was done? Nothing at all. This is not a case of having to accept the inherent dangers of drugs in order to obtain the great benefits. Here is an example of negligence on a nationwide scale. At a minimum, we need ongoing studies of prescribing practices and better tools to help doctors prevent the most common mistakes.

When a physician makes an obvious and serious prescribing error, it is supposed to be caught at the pharmacy—the next link in the safety chain. No one supposes the nation's 170,000 pharmacists can or should second-guess the medical judgment of a doctor. But the pharmacist is supposed to question a prescription that is written for the wrong dose. The pharmacist should question a prescription for penicillin for a patient who is allergic to it. And it is especially important for a pharmacist to question prescriptions for two drugs with a potentially lethal interaction. One such classic danger is the interaction between the antihistamine Hismanal and Nizoral, a drug for fungus infections. The Hismanal manufacturer declares the two drugs should never be prescribed together because of the danger of causing potentially lethal change in the heart rhythm. A team from *U.S. News & World Report* submitted this and two similarly dangerous combination prescriptions to 245 pharmacies in seven cities. Each was a clear-cut case where the pharmacist should have refused to fill the prescription, offered to call the doctor, or sent the patient back to the doctor. However, 32 percent of the pharmacists gave out the two prescriptions. The results "prove the systems to correct prescription drug errors in this country are of very limited reliability," noted Marcus Reidenberg, a pharmacologist at the New York Hospital–Cornell Medical Center. In another survey, Georgetown University pharmacologist and physician Raymond Woosley found that 30 percent of Washington area pharmacies filled prescriptions with another potentially lethal combination, the antihistamine Seldane and the antibiotic erythromycin.[27] With no national monitoring system and few studies in literature, it is impossible to determine the overall risks of pharmacy errors. Worse yet, far-reaching changes are occurring in the field of pharmacy with little thought about the effects on drug safety. Measuring out the medication and preparing the label is a job increasingly done by machine. Pharmacy benefit managers are providing millions of consumers with prescriptions by mail, and monitoring doctors to reduce costs. Workloads on pharmacists are greatly increasing as the number of pills in each prescription is reduced to save money.

In listening to pharmacists discuss their jobs on the Internet, it's easy to see the tremendous pressures of their jobs. "I am a new pharmacist who needs help with ideas for preventing dispensing errors," wrote one young woman. "I find I am making too many mistakes. I think I am making about 1 dispensing error a week. This is causing considerable stress in my life, and it seems the harder I try not to make a mistake, the more mistakes I am making," she noted.

"I did too before I lost my license," responded a colleague. "[Filling] 200 Rx's a day isn't pharmacy, it's factory work." We shouldn't have to listen to the desperate pleas of an overworked, conscientious young woman who wants to do a good job and fears someone will get hurt. We need systems engineered so that a well-trained professional working at normal speed can produce error-free results.

The consumer is the final link in the safety chain. If we were lucky, the bottle in the medicine cabinet would contain a thoroughly tested drug, its dangers and benefits scientifically documented. The pill was manufactured correctly, and is free of glass fragments, or contamination, and will dissolve properly. A knowledgeable doctor made wise use of all the information developed during testing and postmarket surveillance and picked an appropriate drug for the consumer's medical condition. The doctor took the time to discuss the risks and benefits of the drug, and outlined the other choices, including forgoing treatment for now. The pharmacist filled the prescription accurately, while the store computer checked for potentially dangerous drug interactions. The consumer went home with an easy-to-read-and-understand brochure about the drug he or she was going to take. Yet the whole system is of limited use unless the consumer takes the drug as prescribed. In the medical literature can be found abundant evidence that about half the time consumers squander the potential benefits of drugs or needlessly expose themselves to dangers by failing to do so.

In the jargon of medicine, the issue is called "patient compliance," and it is the most extensively researched link in the safety chain. I found 5,723 medical studies published since 1990 in which patient compliance was the subject—or an important element. (While studies of doctor prescribing patterns are few, organized medicine has an intense interest in getting patients to follow instructions.) Drugs were the major focus of these compliance studies, but not the only kind of medical directive considered. One study focused on 26 patients with epilepsy—people who need continuous drug therapy to prevent seizures. The patients got medicine bottles with microprocessors in the caps that recorded every time the bottle was opened. Despite the risk of seizures, one-quarter of the prescribed doses were not taken. The problem, apparently, was remembering to take the drug. Those who needed medication four times a day took only 39 percent of all the doses required. On a once-a-day regimen, however, patients took 87 percent of the prescribed medicine. In this case, the failure to comply had consequences: 7 of 26 patients had seizures after missing one or more doses.[28] Other research shows patients frequently pay a price for failing to take medication as prescribed. For example, in one study 58 percent failed to take a full course of antibiotics for strep throat; as a result almost 1 out of 4 patients had a relapse.[29] Failure to take asthma medication as prescribed is a major cause of preventable emergency room visits and hospitalization in this disorder.[30] Patients are an integral part of the problem of drug safety.

This is the present state of the system that is supposed to minimize the dangers of prescription drugs. From this perspective, serious injuries are not some inevitable price paid to obtain beneficial drugs. Instead, we observe a system filled with lost opportunities to use prescription drugs more safely. In some links of the chain, we see evidence of an unforgivably sloppy system. Why were one-third of pharmacies filling two prescriptions with a potentially lethal interaction? Why did 1 out of 5 doctors prescribe inappropriate drugs for elderly patients? Other lapses, while severe, give us more confidence. Warner-Lambert had major lapses in drug manufacturing, but the company got caught and was compelled to act. The most troubling aspect of the system is the extent to which the whole enterprise flies blind. No one really knows how many people are killed or seriously injured, or how often pharmacists make a dispensing error. Few would suggest a blanket of federal regulation over the prescribing practices of individual physicians. But shouldn't we at least insist on gathering data about the most frequent prescribing errors in order to prevent them? To think about prescription drugs in terms of a safety system is to understand that modern society has been unnecessarily careless about the most dangerous thing we do.

CHAPTER EIGHT

Pain

BY 9 A.M. it was already clear that this would be a major event in Washington D.C., a city where a yawn greets an event of merely moderate importance. Just to get a seat, the drug company lobbyists had paid students to stand in line since dawn. In the United States Senate hearing room, the stage had been carefully set to put the heat on the chief witness of the morning. The unfolding drama would star the commissioner of the Food and Drug Administration, David A. Kessler. On this day in February 1996, many members of the United States Senate Committee on Labor were critical of Kessler. A majority supported new legislation that would reduce the FDA's scientific scrutiny of new drugs before approval. They thought the sixteen months it took the FDA to review a new drug application was excessive. To dramatize their point, the senators had arranged a little demonstration at Kessler's expense.

Kessler sat alone at a witness table. In front of him was an

awesome mass of paperwork neatly arranged on two long ta-
bles. Bound in hundreds of separate notebooks with plain
brown cardboard covers were more than 200,000 pages of
documentation. This was all the material submitted to the
FDA about the testing of a single new drug. To those who
understood the potential dangers of drugs, an independent review of the complete scientific record might seem reasonable.
But for the television cameras that would compress this scene
into a ten-second spot, it would create exactly the impression
that the committee majority intended. Kessler would have
to testify while appearing to be buried in a mountain of
paperwork.

The chairman, Kansas Republican Senator Nancy Kassebaum, explained this was the documentation required to get
FDA approval for a new drug.

"This is for aspirin?" joked Senator Barbara Mikulski, a
Democrat from Maryland. She got a big laugh.

"It may have been, when aspirin was presented," said
Kassebaum.

"You couldn't get aspirin approved today," said Mikulski.[1]

The senator unwittingly picked a perfect example for exploring the performance of the drug safety system. Aspirin and
other nonsteroidal anti-inflammatory drugs provide such effective pain relief that they rank among the most widely used
drugs in the world.*

However, these drugs are so hazardous in long-term use that
in the United States they send about as many people to the
hospital every year as do all auto accidents.[2] In Britain, anti-
inflammatory drugs account for 25 percent of all adverse
reactions reported over a ten-year period, the worse results

---

*This class of medicines will be referred to simply as "anti-inflammatory drugs." The term
"nonsterodial" is used to distinguish them from cortisone and similar systemic drugs.

for any class of drug.[3] In 1995, over-the-counter Aleve (naproxen) caused more adverse reactions reported to the FDA than any other drug in the United States, prescription or over-the-counter.[4] If any drugs deserve to be tested so thoroughly that the results create a scientific record thousands of pages long, anti-inflammatory drugs should lead the list. As one World Health Organization official put it, "The history of anti-inflammatory drug therapy is littered with failures resulting from unanticipated and unacceptable toxicity."[5] Thirteen of these drugs had to be hastily withdrawn because they were too toxic—setting a worldwide record for drug testing failure.[6] Even the surviving drugs had risks so serious that every patient should get a clear and understandable warning. Despite millions of dollars spent on advertising to tell people about these drugs, few learn the truth about the risks that they are taking until disaster strikes. This is exactly what happened to a Chicago corporate lawyer named James Morton.

Only a few weeks before the Senate hearing, James Morton lay alone at dawn in a hospital room in Evanston, Illinois. To sustain his life, the fifty-five-year-old Morton was connected to a nightmarish maze of plastic tubing. In the front of his pelvis, a tube had been inserted into the abdominal cavity to drain the pus and fluid from his body's battle with a raging infection. Farther up his abdomen were two more drain tubes near other sites where bacteria had also festered and multiplied. Additional IV lines were inserted for the antibiotics to fight infection, and to provide nutrition. Despite this mass of tubing, Morton was gradually losing a little more ground to the infection every day.

Just after 6:30 A.M. one January morning, a troop of thirty specialists, residents, and medical students crowded into Morton's room. He was an interesting case for this teaching hospital. Without the aggressive medical interventions for which modern hospitals are famous, Morton would surely die. But with deft use of the powerful tools available, they had a good chance to save him. Trillions of dangerous bacteria and other microorganisms normally live an uneventful life in the stomach, intestine, and colon. They are tightly contained by membrane barriers that admit to the body only selected nutrients and fluids. In Morton's case, the bacteria had breached this critical defensive barrier and were now multiplying inside the normally sterile abdominal cavity, a location where the body is not well equipped to combat infection.

On this cold Midwest winter morning, Morton's case was especially interesting to the assembled physicians. A diagnostic test now provided the answer to the baffling question that had plagued them all week. The repeated infusion of the most powerful antibiotics in the medical arsenal had not beaten back the infection. In fact, Morton had gotten slowly worse. But the day before, a specialist had examined the walls of Morton's stomach through an endoscope, a flexible, optical tube that can be threaded down the throat. Pictures taken through the endoscope now explained why Morton was getting worse instead of better. A small hole in his stomach continued to leak bacteria to renew the infection. The obvious solution was surgery to stop the leak. But the infection had already taken such a toll on Morton's previous robust health that the surgeons thought surgery was too risky. For the assembled doctors, it was a challenging medical problem, planning how to build up Morton's health for surgery while holding the infection at bay. For Morton, it was possibly the worse, most painful week in his entire life. This dire medical crisis had been created by an anti-inflammatory drug that is similar to aspirin.

Morton's experience is an appallingly common event today.

Every year anti-inflammatory drugs cause the hospitalization of approximately 70,000 people for perforated ulcers or severe gastrointestinal bleeding.[7] The most callous may shrug and say that maybe this is the price we pay for having effective painkillers that benefit millions of people. However, a closer look reveals a flawed safety system that doesn't protect consumers. Morton was a case in point.

Sixteen months earlier, Morton had a medical problem that often afflicts athletic middle-aged men. Morton had developed a minor but persistent pain in his right arm, blamed on his golf swing. While not severe, it did bother him when he wrote comments on legal briefs or carried his briefcase. An orthopedist told him the problem was an inflamed tendon. Among the treatments he provided was a prescription for an anti-inflammatory drug called Oruvail. It is the same drug as the over-the-counter Orudis KT, except at a higher dose in sustained-release tablets taken once a day. For Morton, the drug worked. The pain went away, and if he skipped a day, it often came back. After taking Oruvail for fifteen months, he experienced intense stomach pains one Sunday morning. They were so severe that he rushed to the nearest hospital emergency room. After surgery to repair the perforated ulcer, he went home. But instead of getting better, he got worse. The endoscope examination showed that the original surgery was flawed and had left the stomach leaking its contents into the abdominal cavity. When this was finally discovered, James Morton's survival was by no means a sure thing. In fact, about 1 out of 10 patients do not survive a severe perforated ulcer or gastrointestinal bleeding episode caused by anti-inflammatory drugs. Overall, these drugs kill more than 7,000 people every year.[8] Fortunately, Morton not only survived, he fully recovered. He continues to play golf regularly and does not use anti-inflammatory drugs.

But the Morton case illustrates a break- down in several key links in the safety chain.

Oruvail had been tested thoroughly enough that the manufacturer, Wyeth-Ayerst Laboratories, knew it could cause perforated ulcers and severe bleeding. However, similar drugs were widely used for seventy-five years before these hazards were fully understood. Without systematic testing, even severe and frequent adverse effects may not be noticed for decades. The ability of even lethal side effects to escape detection is a special problem of drugs. If the designers of an airplane or ocean liner overlook some key safety issue, the shortcoming will become painfully evident when the vehicle crashes or sinks. As the history of aspirin shows, critical drug defects may remain invisible for many years.

Aspirin was the first major anti-inflammatory drug. It is a direct chemical descendant of willow bark and wintergreen oil, which are among the oldest known remedies for arthritis pain. The active ingredient in these early medicines was salicylic acid. It was so corrosive that it could also be used to remove warts and bunions. By the nineteenth century, a milder chemical relative called sodium salicylate was used to treat rheumatism. However, its taste, described by users as "disgusting," made it unpopular. Aspirin emerged from the chemical search for the rheumatism remedy without the horrible taste. By chance, the small chemical change that improved the taste helped make acetylsalicylic acid one of the most effective anti-inflammatory drugs ever discovered. After languishing on the shelf of the Bayer chemical company for several decades, it became a best-seller soon after it was first marketed at the beginning of this century. While its value in fevers, arthritis, and muscle pain was quickly recognized, it took seventy years to appreciate its capacity to cause life-threatening ulcers and internal bleeding.

Anti-inflammatory drugs block the swelling and inflammation that are an integral part of the body's natural response to tissue injury. According to the most widely accepted theory, this response is triggered in part by short-haul chemical messengers called prostaglandins.[9] At the site of an injury, prostaglandins are released and trigger a complex cascade of events in the nearby area. Unlike hormones, which circulate throughout the body, prostaglandins are active only in the immediate area where they are released.[10] Anti-inflammatory drugs block the formation of prostaglandins and therefore stop this chemical cascade of events at the site of injury. That is how they prevent inflammation. Unfortunately, prostaglandins do other jobs in the human body as well. In the kidneys, they help regulate chloride levels. In the developing fetus, they help maintain the proper blood circulation through the fetal heart.

However, hundreds of thousands of people end up in the hospital because prostaglandins have another important task. They help maintain the vital protective coating of the stomach and duodenum, the link between the stomach and the small intestine.[11] To prevent damage to the stomach wall, the cells maintain a protective coating of mucus and acid-neutralizing bicarbonate of soda. Anti-inflammatory drugs block the chemical message that tells the stomach cells to secrete the protective coating. This is the inescapable limitation of present anti-inflammatory drugs. The same chemical messenger that triggers painful inflammation also manages the protection of the stomach and duodenum. Blocking the chemical messenger impairs both functions.[12] Many anti-inflammatory drugs can damage the stomach in a second way. They are themselves acids that can further irritate the intestinal tissue. Enteric pill coatings, or taking the tablet with food, can sometimes reduce this part of the risk.

Even prescribing physicians often underestimate how rapidly and how severely anti-inflammatory drugs damage the gastrointestinal tract. For example, researchers used an endoscope to examine the stomach of eighty-two arthritis patients taking aspirin for three months or more.[13] Seventy-five percent had reddened, damaged areas, 40 percent had gastric erosions, and 20 percent had outright bleeding ulcers. These results were compared to untreated controls of similar age. Among those who did not take aspirin, none had ulcers and only 5 percent had reddened areas of the stomach lining. Most newer anti-inflammatory drugs are just as dangerous as aspirin—and by some measures, more toxic.[14] After six months of treatment, medically significant stomach or intestinal damage was seen in 61 percent of the patients taking Orudis, in 37 percent taking ibuprofen (Advil, Motrin) and 29 percent of those on Voltaren.[15] These adverse effects may appear within weeks. After one month of treatment, ulcers were found in 10 percent of the patients taking Feldene and 9 percent of those taking naproxen.[16]

Sometimes the first warning sign of gastrointestinal tract damage for those taking anti-inflammatory drugs is heartburn or some similar stomach upset. As warning signs go, this is of limited use since episodes of heartburn can be so frequent and have so many other causes. However, if the pain persists, the next stop is the doctor's office. A story of arthritis patients showed that in roughly one year's time, 25 percent sought medical attention for stomach pain or related problems.[17] The more dangerous outcomes are a stomach ulcer, a more severe perforated ulcer, and major gastrointestinal bleeding. These events occur in 2 to 4 percent of those who take anti-inflammatory drugs for one year.[18] A perforated ulcer or GI bleed is a life-threatening emergency and often comes without any warning symptoms. A British surgeon studied 141 cases so severe that the patients died or required emergency surgery.[19] He found that 58 percent had no prior warning symptoms. James Morton's experience in Evanston, Illinois, was typical, not unusual. These adverse effects of anti-inflammatory drugs are so common and so severe that they play a large role in the overall cost of treating arthritis. One research estimated that treatment of the adverse effects of anti-inflammatory drugs accounted for one-third of the $12 billion annual cost of arthritis.[20] In another study, the use of anti-inflammatory drugs doubled the annual Medicare bills of arthritis patients—mostly for hospital treatment of the drug complications.[21]

These are the basic facts about a family of drugs now in use for the better part of a century. What lessons does this teach about the system for minimizing the number of deaths and serious injuries from prescription drugs? Surely the anti-inflammatory drug experience emphasizes the pivotal role of drug testing in safety. Aspirin was sold for seventy years without an understanding of the major gastrointestinal hazards of its original use—for long-term relief of arthritis. Even as late as 1974, a pharmacologist writing a history of aspirin confidently proclaimed, "The number of side effects is few and the number of deaths approaches an irreducible level."[22] Without systematic study and testing, major hazards of drugs may continue undetected for decades. Critics of the present system have often asked, How many people die while waiting for new drugs to be tested and approved? The answer: Many fewer than if an undetected hazard harms people for decades. As it happened, the anti-inflammatory drugs marketed to compete with aspirin were better tested, but it soon became apparent that testing was still not rigorous enough.

Anti-inflammatory drugs created the second major postwar drug-testing crisis. In 1962, the thalidomide tragedy was the wake-up call, warning that powerful new wonder drugs also carried great risks. It resulted in most of the advanced western nations requiring formal clinical trials for new drugs, and independent government panels to evaluate the results. As a result, the new anti-inflammatory drugs moving toward the marketplace in the late 1970s and early 1980s were much more extensively tested. They were given to animals for two years to check for cancer risk and overall toxicity. Each drug was compared to aspirin in randomized clinical trials in which the patients were carefully monitored. The results were scrutinized by experts in pharmacology, medicine, and biostatistics. Despite these precautions, a major fiasco still occurred.

In the United States, Oraflex, Suprol, and Zomax were withdrawn; in Britain, Prinalgin, Dytransin, Flenac, Feprazone, and Flosint; in Spain, Pacyl and Rengasil, in France, Pixifenide and Pirprofen.[23] In all, thirteen approved anti-inflammatory drugs were withdrawn for safety reasons. In the wake of the thaliodmide tragedy, most nations had also set up early warning systems so doctors could rapidly report suspected adverse reactions. With the introduction of the new anti-inflammatory drugs, the systems were loaded with distress signals. Zomax could cause potentially lethal allergic reactions. Suprol damaged the kidneys. Oraflex harmed the liver and the kidneys. Flenac caused ugly skin eruptions. So what went wrong? Although testing revealed potential dangers in all of these drugs, the drug approval authorities were still reluctant to reject a drug.

The case of Oraflex provides a bizarre case in point. Oraflex was an expensive competitor for aspirin, readily approved in both Britain and the United States. Yet in testing, clear evidence emerged that Oraflex caused the skin to become supersensitive to the sun. Exposure to a few hours of direct sun could result in rash in about 10 percent of the patients, and caused the fingernails to separate from the nail bed in another 10 percent.[24] In arguing that these problems should not bar approval, the manufacturer Eli Lilly noted that in many cases the nail only separated about half the way down; it did not fall off altogether. The company also suggested that consumers apply opaque nail polish for protection. This crazy idea is a testament to the safety priorities of a pharmaceutical company with millions invested in a new drug. Eli Lilly actually marketed an alternative to aspirin that required users to apply protective nail polish before going outdoors. For the drug approval authorities, however, Oraflex did provide a dilemma. When was it time to say a drug had just one adverse effect too many? It was easier to judge efficacy. There was a procedure—a clinical trial—and a set of reasonably clear rules to decide whether or not a drug had the stated medical effect. Toxicity was harder to judge. Since all modern drugs have side effects, how many adverse effects were too many? Drugs for major clinical depression trigger so many unpleasant side effects that about 15 percent of the people decide the drug is worse than the disease.[25] Drugs for cancer treatment cause debilitating side effects in almost everyone treated. In such a world of drug toxicity, where does a partially separated fingernail rank?

As it turned out, however, Oraflex did have one side effect too many, by almost any measure. Oraflex was particularly long-lived in the body. While ibuprofen was broken down in about two hours, Oraflex remained active for almost a full day. In elderly patients who eliminated almost all drugs more slowly, Oraflex could build up to concentrations that sometimes proved toxic to the kidneys and liver and lethal to the patient. Oraflex was approved in the United States in April 1982. By August, at least 30 deaths were reported to the FDA, and the drug was withdrawn. Lilly was later prosecuted criminally for failing to report to the FDA information about many similar cases occurring abroad.[26] An investigation by Congress revealed that the drug might never have been approved in the United States if the European deaths had been promptly reported as required by law.

In 1988, a Stanford medical professor named James Fries wrote a medical journal editorial making an important point about the drug withdrawals. Fries pointed out that all the attention was focusing on the newly discovered side effects. The important danger, he noted, was thousands upon thousands of perforated ulcers and episodes of severe intestinal bleeding that were being caused by all the drugs in the anti-inflammatory family.[27] To save lives and make the system safe, this central problem of gastrointestinal damage still had to be faced.

There were efforts to find solutions. One was a new drug called misoprostol, or Cytotec. When taken with anti-inflammatory drugs, it could reduce the incidence of ulcers by nearly 40 percent.[28] But at the recommended dose, it also caused diarrhea in 14 to 40 percent of the patients. Also, something bothered practitioners about giving a drug with its own obvious GI side effects to reduce other GI side effects. So it did not become first-line therapy for anyone taking anti-inflammatory drugs over the long term. A more frequent solution was the much more easily tolerated drugs for ulcers, such as Tagamet, Pepcid, and Zantac. It was a seemingly logical solution—a powerful and effective anti-ulcer drug for people who developed ulcers from their anti-inflammatory medication. However, in 1996 a long-term study from Stanford Medical School researchers provided troubling evidence that the ulcer drug solution might be a serious medical mistake.[29] While the ulcer drugs relieved the immediate stomach pains, they appeared to double the risk of a life-threatening perforated ulcer or GI bleed. As this is written, hopes for a solution ride on a new generation of anti-inflammatory drugs. They are believed to block the prostaglandins involved in inflammation but leave unaffected those involved in protecting the stomach. Early results presented at scientific meetings show less damage to the stomach. However, two of the first five drugs to enter human testing have already been abandoned for toxicity; the fate of the others is yet to be determined.

In the meantime, the safest strategy is to prescribe anti-inflammatory drugs only when absolutely necessary and to warn consumers about the risks they take. Some people with arthritis or rheumatism can get adequate relief from acetaminophen (or Tylenol), a pain reliever without anti-inflammatory effects both beneficial and harmful. It should be the first choice.[30] Other patients—for whom these drugs are routinely prescribed without careful assessment—don't need long-term treatment with any drug. In one British study of arthritis, patients sometimes got a palcebo instead of an active drug. About 40 percent of the patients switched to a placebo didn't even notice any difference. Another study dramatically illustrated how often the drugs were used unnecessarily. Among a group of elderly patients whose prescriptions were reviewed at a hospital, 11 percent said they did not know why they were taking anti-inflammatory drugs and another 31 percent said the drugs provided no benefit.[31] After the anti-inflammatory drugs were stopped in this group, one-third noticed no symptoms requiring a painkiller. While billions are spent every year to advertise and promote wider use of anti-inflammatory drugs, there are almost no programs to discourage overmedication or inappropriate use of drugs.

Sanford Roth, an arthritis specialist with a long interest in the hazards of these drugs, noted, "Industry was understandably not anxious to pursue silent ghosts when their products were so expensively produced and popularly received in the marketplace."[32]

By 1988—only eight decades after the introduction of aspirin—the FDA and the medical community finally began to face the central problem that remained unsolved—the gastrointestinal tract hazards. How was the nation's drug safety system to respond to a new understanding of major health hazards of a very successful and popular family of drugs? No one was suggesting withdrawing aspirin and ibuprofen from the market. But how should a major threat endangering 13 million people be managed? The first step seems obvious. Every consumer taking these drugs for the long term ought to have a clear and unmistakable warning about the risks involved. However, this clashed directly with a medical doctrine that lay behind the willingness of so many million Americans to take so many powerful drugs: Don't scare the consumers. To sound a warning loud enough to be heard by the millions of elderly patients taking anti-inflammatory drugs might create nationwide alarm. At the very least, it would generate embarrassing questions about the previous vigilance of doctors, the drug companies, and the FDA. On the other hand, it would be unfair to imply that the health establishment would ignore entirely their moral, ethical, and legal responsibilities.

The result was a compromise that protected the reputations of the authorities but did not threaten the continued sales of these drugs or trigger undue public alarm. A clearly worded warning was indeed issued. **"Serious gastrointestinal toxicity, such as bleeding, ulceration, and perforation, can occur at any time with or without warning symptoms,"** it said. Such problems occurred **"in about 2-4% of patients**

treated for one year." (Boldface in original warning.) Unfortunately, this barely adequate warning was buried in a location where few would see it. It was added to the fine print of the highly technical, densely worded drug disclosure label, a widely available document that is seldom consulted by anyone because of its complex language and unwieldy format. Disclosure labels are not intended to be read by consumers; few alert doctors would likely have time to analyze the fine print, looking for telltale changes between the 1988 and 1989 versions.

To see how ineffectual this step was, let's trace the path of this warning from the disclosure label to James Morton's perforated ulcer. The warning quoted above does appear in the fine print of the Oruvail disclosure label. This information, however, is intended for doctors. For patients, Wyeth Laboratories recommends providing a much less frightening warning. It says:

> Rarely, there are more serious side effects such as gastrointestinal bleeding, which may result in hospitalization and even fatal outcomes.

I do not believe a 2 to 4 percent chance of a serious event is "rare." In fact, the British have proposed describing any risk over 1 percent as "high."[33] The statement was given no special prominence on the label, even though it is the most important and prominent risk of taking the product. But at least it is a warning.

Because of a remarkable loophole in the system, there is no guarantee that consumers actually get the warning that the manufacturer recommends. I couldn't get the warning Morton actually received, but this is the warning my local pharmacy gives to consumers with an Oruvail prescription. All it says is:

Stomach upset is the most common side effect. If this persists or becomes severe, notify your doctor.[34]

By the times James Morton's stomach upset became severe, he was on his way to the emergency room with a perforated ulcer. His doctor had told him nothing of the risks of taking Oruvail continuously for over a year.

Failure to warn consumers about the risks of anti-inflammatory drugs is not an isolated breakdown. As knowledge about the dangers of drugs has grown, the typical solution has been to place a warning on the disclosure label and then forget about it. This was the action taken after it was learned that Hismanal could cause cardiac arrest, that estrogen causes endometrial cancer, that Prozac may cause episodes of mania, that the long-term safety of Ritalin has never been studied, that Felbatol can destroy the bone marrow, that beta-blockers can cause depression, that the blood pressure drug Vasotec can damage the kidneys, that the anticlotting drug Coumadin can cause gangrene, that 4 percent of the people who took the antibiotic Floxin had to discontinue it, as did 15 percent of those who took the antidepressant Zoloft.[35] The response of the FDA and drug companies to the dangers of drugs described throughout this book has been to put a warning in the disclosure label and take little if any further action on the matter. Even when the manufacturer recommends a warning for consumers, the pharmacy may omit it in the printed material for consumers. To insure the public is aware of the documented dangers of drugs might interfere with the relentless drive to sell ever larger numbers of drugs. This is one important reason why safety takes a back seat in the world of prescription drugs.

The story of anti-inflammatory drugs also provides lessons about the overall safety system. It reveals one unique hazard of drugs. Without proper testing, serious hazards may go undetected for decades. Even with rigorous testing, questions about acceptable toxicity may remain because standards of safety are not as clear as the requirement that a drug be effective. When the dangers of anti-inflammatory drugs were fully understood after eighty years of use, the system proved completely inadequate to contain these risks. Thousands of lives could be saved with better information for doctors, elimination of unnecessary and marginal uses, proper warnings to patients and the substitution of safer alternatives whenever possible.

CHAPTER NINE

Sleep

A FORTY-FOUR-YEAR-OLD woman was understandably anxious about the speech she was going to give to two hundred people the next morning. It was the kind of tension that even experienced public speakers often feel. To help her sleep, she took a sleeping pill. It had a dramatic effect. The next thing she knew, it was 12:20 P.M. the next day. She was having lunch and conversing briskly with twelve people she had never met. Later she learned that she had driven to another state and delivered her two-hour lecture illustrated with slides. The sleep medication she had taken was called Halcion.[1]

A thirty-three-year-old woman who was a specialist in brain anatomy appeared at the luggage counter at the airport in Frankfurt, Germany. After an overnight flight from New York, her luggage had not appeared. She was surprised when the airline representative already knew her. The representative also had a completed form in her handwriting. She then boarded a train for Heidelberg, a trip of which she later remembered nothing. To combat the jet lag of the overnight flight, she had taken Halcion.[2]

A Grand Rapids, Michigan, attorney named Stuart Wechsler saw his legal career disintegrate following a six-month bout of depression and hostility. During the same period, he had been taking Halcion because muscle spasms were disrupting his sleep.[3] "It nearly destroyed my career," Wechsler said.

A Texas man named William Freeman erupted in a violent rage and fired a bullet into the brain of his best friend, Donnie Hazelwood, killing him. He had been taking Halcion over a two-and-a-half-year period during which he experienced memory loss, psychotic episodes, paranoia, and other bizarre and unpredictable behavior.[4]

The role of any drug in an unexpected outburst of violence remains complex and controversial. But by 1989, Upjohn had received at least 24 reports of murder, attempted murder, or threatened attack in which Halcion use was apparently associated.[5] The story of Halcion will show how a drug company can undermine the system intended to insure the safety of prescription drugs. With a determined effort, a global giant can neutralize the efforts of concerned doctors, committed government regulators, investigative reporters, and trial lawyers with subpoena power. That is the main lesson of the battle between the Upjohn Company of Kalamazoo, Michigan, and Halcion's critics. (In a 1996 merger with a Swedish firm, the company became Pharmacia & Upjohn and is under new management.) It shows that under some conditions one important danger of a prescription drug can be the company that sells it.

Upjohn was a member of the select club of global pharmaceutical companies that are the most profitable—but by no means the largest—of the world's major industries. For example, the retail giant Wal-Mart has more sales than all ten major U.S. drug companies combined. But Wal-Mart's profits of

$2.7 billion are dwarfed by the drug industry's profits of $17 billion. Of every dollar received by the large drug companies, 16 cents is pure profit. By comparison, auto company profits are only 4 cents on a dollar of sales, tobacco companies 7 cents, oil companies 2 cents. Only about half the major drug companies are headquartered in the United States, but a global comparison produces similar results. The profits of industry, and the reason for these high profits, greatly influence how a company such as Upjohn responds to questions about the safety of a best-selling drug such as Halcion.

It may be the only industry whose profitability can be explained by a single term: the patent. The primary engine of drug industry profitability is the right to patent and sell exclusively a new medicine. If it is a blockbuster, a single patented drug can sustain a multinational drug company for years at a time. Eli Lilly achieved an extraordinary profit margin of 30 cents on the revenue dollar in 1996 largely because of the phenomenal sales of Prozac. The industry gambles millions in a high-stakes lottery to come up with the next blockbuster drug. It is surprising that in hunting the next unique blockbuster the industry often behaves like a herd of cattle, a pack of dogs, or a school of fish, flocking to the same market and opportunity. As a result, the industry has produced 115 different drugs to lower blood pressure and 70 anti-inflammatory drugs.[6] Drugs for depression are the latest target of industry research frenzy with, by one count, 125 different drugs now in development to add to the 30 already approved and on the market.[7] It was in just such a push in the large and important market for sleep aids that Halcion was born.

Behind the walls of the state penitentiary at Jackson, Michigan, stands a special drug-testing facility constructed by the Upjohn Company and a pharmaceutical competitor, Parke-Davis. Known as the Jackson Clinic, it has three twelve-bed wards, a laboratory, and offices for visiting doctors. In May of 1972, a doctor named Harold Oster began a drug study named Protocol 321. He was working for the Upjohn Company, and he was testing a promising new compound that would later be called Halcion. Either the drug or a placebo would be given to carefully selected inmates. The effects of the drug, including any adverse effects, were written down on the case report forms. All this material went over to Upjohn headquarters in Kalamazoo, where the date were coded and analyzed and a technical report written. Oster seldom saw the results. At Upjohn there were three different reviewers to examine the data. It was a careful enough system that it could be expected to work. It took eighteen years to establish beyond question that something had gone badly wrong in Protocol 321.

In the year 1972, Halcion was a promising new candidate for what was then the hottest new class of drugs affecting the human brain and behavior. They are called benzodiazepines and include tranquilizers such as Valium and Librium, and sleep aids such as Restoril, Doral, and Dalmane. By the late 1980s, benzodiazepines were taken by 7 percent of the United States population in a year's time, about 10 million people. The drug texts assert that all the benzodiazepines are quite similar in their calming and sedative effect on the human brain.[8] Halcion, however, seemed to have two other characteristics that separated it from the pack. It was especially potent and therefore achieved its effect at lower doses.[9] Also, it acted quickly and disappeared quickly.[10] This fast-acting profile might make it an ideal sleep aid. It would bring sleep rapidly and largely disappear by the next morning. The subject would not feel groggy or hungover as sometimes occurred with Restoril. But an unusually potent, fast-acting mind drug also had substantial risks. It might well be addictive, to have withdrawal effects, and to cause aberrant behavior. To make sure that the benefits outweigh the risks is what drug testing is all about. That was taking place in the penitentiary in Jackson.

For forty-two days the prisoners took Halcion, starting with a dose of 1 mg—the highest Upjohn envisioned for the new drug. The side effects were terrible. The 30 patients on the active drug experienced a total of 453 adverse effects, including memory loss, depression, paranoia, and euphoria.[11] The 1 mg dose was so toxic that it was discontinued partway into the study and a 0.5 mg dose substituted for 8 subjects. In all, psychiatric adverse effects appeared in 50 percent of the patients taking Halcion.[12] Such a toxicity profile could have either spelled the immediate termination of Halcion's future as a useful drug—or resulted in research being started over from scratch to determine whether the drug was safer and still useful at much lower doses.

These were not the results reported when the data were tabulated at Upjohn headquarters. The summary merely noted that 7 of 30 patients on the active drug appeared to have psychiatric side effects compared to 3 of 20 on placebo. Given the smaller number of patients on placebo, this was virtually a clean bill of health. The discrepancy has never been fully explained.[13] However, the clinical testing at Upjohn was tainted with outright fraud. William Franklin of Houston, an internal medicine specialist who worked on five later Halcion studies, admitted fabricating laboratory test results. A Vicksburg, Mississippi, psychiatrist named Samuel Feurst conducted the major long-term clinical study of Halcion. The FDA disqualified Fuerst from all future drug testing work after investigators determined he apparently did not give the drug to patients.[14] An FDA investigator later declared, "Some of the fraud appeared to be so obvious that it would be difficult to overlook."[15]

Upjohn's scientific case that Halcion was safe and that it effectively helped people get to sleep included this kind of evidence. In 1977, it won approval to sell the drug in the Netherlands at the 1 mg dose that proved so toxic among the Michigan prisoners. The results were just what one might expect. The first evidence of trouble came from a Dutch psychiatrist, Cees van der Kroef. After nine months of observing patients he became convinced the drug caused psychiatric problems. In a letter to the *Lancet*, a British medical journal with a worldwide audience, van der Kroef listed twenty-seven different adverse reactions to Halcion, including paranoid reactions, suicidal tendencies, aggression, and continuous fear of going insane.[16] A similar article in a Dutch medical journal was picked up by local television and newspapers.

With Halcion just approved in Britain and not yet on the market in the United States, van der Kroef's safety concerns were a threat to the future of this fledgling drug. Upjohn did not delay in mounting a counterattack. The company convened a group of ten medical experts and ethicists in Boston and persuaded them to write a reply to the *Lancet*. Claiming to have "reviewed the data" on Halcion safety, the group wrote in the *Lancet* that "our findings do not substantiate van der Kroef's letter."[17] In a peculiar twist of logic, the writers said that if the adverse effects were real, then they probably were the result of the high 1 mg dose. (In the law, this is like claiming you didn't rob the store, but if you did, it was only because you were forced to do it.) The letter appeared to be an effective rebuttal from a group of specialists from the United States, Canada, and Holland. However, an FDA investigation later concluded "there was minimal review of the clinical data" and that specialists got "only selective data."[18] The lead author of the attack on van der Kroef conceded later in a television interview that the group had been duped by Upjohn.[19]

The next assault on van der Kroef came a few months later from a prominent United States drug researcher named Louis Lasagna. To impeach van der Kroef, Lasagna resorted to tactics that are usually the last refuge of embattled politicians—blame the news media. He wrote a "Point of View" article for the *Lancet* entitled "Trial by Media." Most of the article was devoted to revealing that the Dutch news media had publicized van der Kroef's concerns. Lasagna likely realized that doctors take a dislike to news reports that alarm their patients. "The public should demand ethical behavior from journalists," Lasagna proclaimed. However, Lasagna did not disclose to *Lancet* readers that he had worked with Upjohn. The two attacks on van der Kroef set an ugly pattern that would be repeated many times in the years to come. Because Halcion was a dangerous drug, physicians would speak out about its dangers. Sensing a threat to its market, Upjohn would seek to attack its critics.

Back in Kalamazoo, Upjohn must have realized that the international furor was not going to make it any easier to win FDA approval to market Halcion in the United States. As one top Upjohn official wrote: "If my sources are anywhere near correct, the FDA will *never* approve Halcion without tremendous pressure. We have the people willing to exert the pressure but we must orchestrate it."[20] As it happened, Upjohn was fortunate that a key figure at the FDA over many years' time apparently never wavered from a firmly held position that Halcion was a safe drug. His name was Paul Leber, a medical doctor who was director of the Division of Neuropharmacological Drug Products. FDA commissioners come and go, and hold most of the press conferences. To this day Leber has remained the FDA's senior official for mind- and behavior-altering drugs. He, and his immediate superior in drug evaluation, had the final say about all such drugs. If Upjohn needed a sympathetic ear at the FDA, it could find no more strategically placed expert than the head of neuropharmacological drugs. Over the years to come, Leber would back Halcion despite the objections of his own medical reviewer, concerns from FDA safety monitors, numerous critical magazine and television stories, and petitions from outside experts.

In the year 1982, however, the person at the FDA who was supposed to know the most about Halcion was the medical reviewer in Leber's division. Her name was Theresa Woo. She had serious doubts about Halcion's safety since she first reviewed the clinical data back in 1977. She had declared back then that Halcion was "not approvable" because it was five times more likely to cause anmesia than another chemically similar sleep aid and fifteen times more likely than placebo.[21] However, approval was delayed for another five years for other reasons, and it was not until 1982 that the revived Halcion application landed back at the FDA. Woo was still concerned about Halcion's safety, but was opposed by her boss, Paul Leber. He discounted the most serious episodes of bizarre behavior as resulting from the high 1 mg dose allowed in the Netherlands, and thought the other adverse effects were common to the whole family of drugs.[22]

Leber's backing meant Halcion was probably headed for approval. However, a critical issue remained. Woo, still concerned about the safety of Halcion, wanted the label instructions for Halcion to limit it to fourteen days' use. There was substantial scientific evidence to support Woo's concern. Using Halcion for more than a few days was a kind of pact with the devil that could extract a heavy price when the subject stopped taking it. The effect is called rebound insomnia. For example, one study showed that for about five days, total sleep time improved. By fifteen days, the effects were sharply reduced as the subject developed tolerance to the drug. When the drug was discontinued, the insomnia was much worse than before.[23] Addiction, seizures, and other adverse effects could appear with long-term use. Woo won this battle, and the FDA proposed label instructions that would recommend only fourteen days of use.

At Upjohn, the fourteen-day limit was greeted with great concern. "A 14-day limit could reduce projected sales by 50% over a 10 year period," noted one Upjohn official.[24] The company decided to press revised product labeling despite the safety risks. An FDA investigation concluded ten years later, "Some ex-employees we interviewed openly stated that this drug was totally inappropriate for long-term use and key people at Upjohn knew it."

Nevertheless, Upjohn pressed for a change in the label instructions that would permit long-term use—and won. When first approved, the warning on Halcion's label instructions merely suggested that physicians prescribe only a one-month supply.[25]

The most tragic cases in which Halcion was alleged to be involved included long-term use. This would include two cases cited earlier—Freeman, who put a bullet in his best friend's brain, and Ilo Grundberg, who put eight bullets into her sleeping, eighty-three-year-old mother.

At the FDA, Theresa Woo remained responsible for monitoring Halcion. After two years on the market in the United States, she was still concerned. She went to Leber and suggested that the Halcion disclosure label ought to have a warning about the frequent adverse effects on the central nervous system. She noted that the FDA had received many adverse reaction reports of hallucinations, sleepwalking, confused states, and depersonalization. Leber objected, citing some of the problems involved in interpreting spontaneous anecdotal reports, the limitations noted in an earlier chapter. However, Leber did suggest that the issue be referred to the FDA's specialists in adverse reaction reporting at the Division of Pharmacoviligance and Epidemiology.[26] Thus, in 1985 the Halcion question landed on the desks of two FDA drug safety specialists, Diane K. Wysowski and David Barash. The two examined every adverse reaction report received for Halcion and compared it to those for other benzodiazepine sleep aids. For example, Wysowski collected all the adverse reaction reports mentioning bizarre behavior. She found 59 for Halcion but just 2 for Restoril. She totaled up the cases of "confusion." For Halcion, 133 reports, for Restoril, just 2. The results for amnesia were similar—106 versus 3. Thus Wysowski and Barash became convinced that Halcion was much more dangerous than other sleep aids.

When Wysowski and Barash's data reinforced Theresa Woo's concerns, Paul Leber was still not persuaded. He rejected the findings as unscientific, triggering a bitter internal battle that would continue for years until Wysowski and Barash were finally allowed to publish their analysis in a medical journal.[27] One of the weaknesses of the FDA system is that the division responsible for monitoring the safety of drugs in the marketplace must take its findings back to the official who approved the drug in the first place. Not only was Leber unmovable regarding the safety of Halcion, the FDA system had no mechanism for getting a fresh, independent look at the question.

Meanwhile, in Kalamazoo the Upjohn management still had to deal with a worldwide chorus of concern about the safety of Halcion. Inside the company, the drug-monitoring staff was seeing the same flood of adverse reaction reports that had triggered Wysowski's concerns at the FDA. (In fact, experience in Britain and Holland was similar to that in the United States.) Some Upjohn staff members were worried. Critics emerged in several countries. In Holland, van der Kroef continued to be concerned about Halcion; in Britain, psychiatrist Ian Oswald published a paper critical of Halcion safety; in the United States, Anthony Kales of the Pennsylvania State College of Medicine became a public critic. The published data from experts with credentials in the field—and the personal experience of writers and reporters who took Halcion—triggered a wave of news media reports critical of Halcion. The famous novelist William Styron wrote a moving account of his depression, triggered in part by Halcion. A California writer named Cynthia Ehrlich wrote a dramatic account of inexplicable fears and paranoia.

Upjohn management responded on two fronts. Inside the company, those who were critical of Halcion were gradually pushed out, often with early-retirement agreements.[28] This apparently included officials who managed the clinical reporting system or worked on drug safety evaluation. To meet outside concerns, Upjohn formed a committee to combat its critics. According to the FDA investigation report, "This committee vigorously sought to suppress the publication of unfavorable studies and attempted to silence Halcion critics."

One of the company's targets was the British psychiatrist Ian Oswald. When he sent a paper about Halcion to the *Archives of General Psychiatry*, a cooperative editor who had been an Upjohn consultant showed a copy to Upjohn. After Upjohn objected, the paper was rejected. The committee also successfully blocked the publication of a critical study in the *New England Journal of Medicine*.[29] An FDA investigator would conclude that the committee also supplied false, misleading, or inaccurate information to government regulatory agencies and to its own consultants who were helping Upjohn defend Halcion.[30] According to one employee who left, the atmosphere inside Upjohn was to "defend the product at all costs."[31]

Nevertheless, by the year 1989 it still looked like Upjohn might be in serious trouble. It had survived adverse news reports, defeated the concerns of safety regulators, and blocked the publication of some critical studies. This time, however, the Halcion battleground was going to be a court of law. Normally, it is quite difficult for someone severely injured to recover damages from a drug company. If the adverse effect is mentioned in the disclosure label, the consumer is deemed to have been warned about the danger.[32] While ignorance of the law is no excuse for a criminal act, ignorance of a drug's adverse effects can be an acceptable defense in a product liability action. Under some circumstances a company can admit that its drug might have caused harm but that it was unaware of the danger. Therefore, one of the few ways to recover damages from a drug company is to prove that it knew about a drug's danger but failed to act. In such lawsuits, the injured party may subpoena a drug company's internal records to determine just what it did and did not know about the dangers of a particular drug. This makes product liability lawsuits enormously expensive, because experts must comb through tens of thousands of pages of often cryptic internal documents, case reports, and medical records. But if a determined lawyer has expert help, it can be done.

In Salt Lake City, Utah, Ilo Marie Gundberg had filed a $21 million lawsuit charging that adverse effects of Halcion had caused her to shoot her mother in 1988. In support of that lawsuit, thousands of pages of Upjohn documents had been produced. Another difficulty in product liability lawsuits is locating a suitably knowledgeable and courageous expert who is willing under any circumstances to testify against a drug company or another doctor. However, in this case one of the victims of Upjohn's campaign to discredit its critics—Ian Oswald—was willing to work on the case. Among the documents that Upjohn had to produce were the original case reports for the 1972 study at the penitentiary at Jackson, Michigan. Oswald spent one thousand hours going through the Upjohn records. He was so careful and systematic that he spotted the large discrepancy between the 423 adverse effects on the case report forms and the clean bill of health suggested by tabulated results submitted to the FDA. Oswald had found the proverbial smoking gun. Upjohn's own early study implicated the drug.

Upjohn, however, would use a well-practiced strategy that drug companies routinely employ to suppress evidence about how the company handled safety concerns and the harm their products do to consumers. It would quickly settle the lawsuit. In return for damage payments, the company would require that the victims say nothing about the amount paid. By avoiding a public trial, drug companies can also avoid disclosure of any of their documents, often winning a specific court order sealing the documents and blocking their use in other lawsuits.

That is what Upjohn did in 1991, and the amount of the damages paid to Ilo Marie Grundberg has never been disclosed. While these legal tactics can typically control the actions of lawyers, they could not quite contain this explosive situation. It quickly became known around the world that vital evidence about Halcion was under seal in a Salt Lake City courthouse. The British Medicines Control Agency demanded that Upjohn produce the revised results of Protocol 321 and other testing data. After a review, the British ordered Halcion withdrawn from the market.

The British action and the discovery of Protocol 321 triggered still another safety crisis for Halcion. The furor included a front-page article in the *New York Times*, a major story in *Newsweek*, and programs on the BBC's *Panarama* and CBS's *60 Minutes*. In most of the coverage, the basic elements were the same: interviews with Ian Oswald and other prominent critics, frightening stories from people who had taken Halcion, and in some accounts the results of Protocol 321. In response to the public outcry, the FDA announced it would investigate Upjohn.

In a high-profile response, Upjohn announced it would sue its most prominent critic, Ian Oswald, for libel. And so began still another cycle of criticism and counterattack. Upjohn chose its next battlefield carefully. The company might have met its critics in open court in the Grundberg case. Oswald and others were going to testify as expert witnesses. But the company had settled with an agreement that barred the disclosure of the evidence about Protocol 321. Instead, it chose to attack the strongest statement Oswald had made in a public forum, a comment in the *New York Times* characterizing Upjohn's behavior as "one long fraud." But Upjohn did not sue the *New York Times* for libel in the United States—where a more permissive legal doctrine on defamation encourages a robust public debate. Instead, it sued Oswald under the strict English libel laws, even though the *New York Times* does not publish an edition in Britain.[33] English law is so sensitive to the nuances of words that cast aspersions on character that one music critic's publisher paid £10,000 in damages for an offhand comment that a raspy-voiced performer "couldn't sing." (She could sing, and gave concerts.) Upjohn also sued the BBC for the *Panorama* program.

The result was a protracted lawsuit in which each side spent more than $1 million on legal fees. When a judgment came down in 1994, the results would be disappointing to anyone concerned about the safety of Halcion, and how Upjohn handled the question. A British judge concluded Upjohn and Oswald libeled each other. Compared to the legal fees, the awards were small: Upjohn had to pay Oswald $75,000 and Oswald was to pay Upjohn $37,500. Oswald also had to pay damages to an Upjohn official he accused of "lying," and the BBC had to pay Upjohn $90,000 damages for its *Panorama* program. The judge concluded that Upjohn had made "serious errors and omissions" and in some cases behaved in a "reckless" manner. But he was not persuaded that Upjohn officials lied (that is, made knowingly false statements) or deliberately concealed information (a fraud). The next investigator, however, was not so kind to Upjohn.

An FDA investigative team led by the Detroit District's D. Michael Erpsamer descended on Upjohn headquarters in

December of 1991. They interviewed present and former employees, obtained the original records for Protocol 321, and began to compare Upjohn's internal records with what was submitted to the FDA. After three months' work, the investigators made some preliminary findings. "We conclude the firm has engaged in an ongoing pattern of misconduct with Halcion," their report said.[34] However, in March 1992 the FDA team was abruptly ordered to discontinue the investigation. On the exact day Erpsamer was ordered off the case, he had also gotten a call from Upjohn telling him a new batch of records he had requested for the investigation were ready to be picked up. "They were extremely important to the investigation," he said. He begged to be allowed to pick up the critical records before closing down the investigation. However, Erpsamer was not allowed to get the records. In June 1996, the agency conceded it had made a mistake by halting the investigation. Citing "management deficiencies," an FDA task force conceded the case should have gone to the Justice Department for a criminal investigation.[35]

When the decidedly mixed verdict was delivered in the Upjohn libel suit against Ian Oswald, the company declared itself the victor. "The company was vindicated," it said.[36] In the larger sense, the company perhaps did triumph over its opponents. Over twenty years, it developed and marketed what proved to be the best-selling benzodiazepine sleep aid. It was not until about 1990 that bad publicity and new competition began to reduce its market share. Upjohn continued to sell Halcion despite the concerns of its own employees, experts in the field, and government drug safety specialists, and despite more than a hundred lawsuits and wave after wave of bad publicity. It was a graphic demonstration of the tremendous power of a global pharmaceutical company. Upjohn had a well-oiled publicity department to get press attention when needed, and skilled and aggressive lawyers who won court orders preventing disclosure of the information it wanted held secret. It could sponsor symposia and pay prominent experts to give testimonials on its behalf. The company was so well connected that it learned in advance about studies with negative results. It could sometimes convince medical journals to reject the manuscripts. Pharmaceutical companies have other major resources not highlighted in this account. They are major contributors to Congress. They typically employ a massive sales force that can make personal contact with a majority of prescribing doctors on a regular basis. Mass mailings, or express packages to hundreds of thousands of physicians, are commonly used to emphasize the company point of view. Repeated studies have shown that most doctors get most of their information about prescription drugs from drug companies.[37] It is a powerful force indeed that in defense of a product can simultaneously take action in the courts, lobby Congress, petition the FDA, bombard the news media, pressure medical journals, and influence doctors. No matter how compelling the underlying facts, a critic's single study, a citizen petition to the FDA, magazine article or book seems puny by comparison.

A policy of defending the product at all costs has been seen in numerous in-depth examinations of drug and medical-device companies. In *Adverse Reactions*, Thomas Maeder found that Parke-Davis just stepped up its advertising to drown out the FDA warnings about the dangers of the antibiotic chloramphenicol.[38] In *Informed Consent*, John A. Byrne reveals how Dow Corning disregarded the concerns of its own employees about silicon gel breast implants.[39] In *At Any Cost*, Morton Mintz shows that A. H. Robins continued to sell the Dalkon Shield contraceptive device even though its own consultants observed life-threatening complications.[40] In my own book *Deadly Medicine*, I revealed that the 3M Company pressed the FDA for wider use of the heart drug Tambocor despite evidence that it could cause cardiac arrest.[41]

Opinions differ, but I personally believe that most of the responsible officials at Upjohn were convinced or convinced themselves that Halcion was no more dangerous than other benzodiazepines. They turned to people inside and outside the company who told them what they wanted to hear. When the spontaneous reports clearly showed that Halcion was more dangerous than its competitors, they declared such data was not reliable. When controlled studies showed Halcion was worse than other sleep aids, they raised other technical objections or concluded they were victims of a vendetta. When the company's own Protocol 321 was found to have omitted most of the adverse effects, Upjohn officials said it was a "transcription error." One of its other studies was so obviously fraudulent that the patient consent forms were all in the doctor's own handwriting. But until FDA investigators spotted the fraud, no one at Upjohn noticed any problems in a study that seemed to show Halcion was safe for long-term use. This process of denial was not unique to Upjohn. In five years of examining evidence about drug safety, I can't recall a single major case without the drug company offering an alibi or technical argument to excuse the unwelcome findings. It is difficult to deny that an airplane crashed, that the money was embezzled, or that the building burned down. It is dangerously easy to deny the early, uncertain warnings about a drug. The system for insuring the safety of prescription drugs is dangerously flawed in leaving so many of these critical judgments to corporations with such well-documented biases.

When denial—a human weakness by no means confined to drug companies—is combined with the global power of a modern integrated pharmaceutical organization, it is a very dangerous situation indeed. The same company owns the laboratories, designs the human studies, tabulates and analyzes the results, gets most of the adverse reaction reports, talks to the doctors, and develops or controls most of the information that is known about a drug. It is too much power concentrated in the hands of the most successful human organization in modern society—a global business. At a time when national governments are being discredited and labor unions severely diminished, the multinational business corporation has been left without peer on the world's stage. Large corporations may be the most adaptable, productive, and efficient organizations yet devised. However, they are unacceptable judges of the safety of prescription drugs. It is a dangerous flaw in the overall system to leave so much of the responsibility for safety in the hands of industry.

CHAPTER TEN

The Doctor's Office

IT'S TIME TO VISIT the doctor's office. Each year the typical American makes about three visits to the doctor, most often to a primary care physician.[1] In more than 700 million annual office visits in the United States, a prescription for a drug is the single most likely outcome. More than a million prescriptions are written every hour of the working day; in a year's time eight prescriptions will be written for every man, woman, and child in the United States.[2] As we all know, doctors are busy. So office visits are short. Two-thirds are less than fifteen minutes, including one-third that last under ten minutes.[3] For all the millions spent testing and evaluating new drugs, the safety of prescription drugs depends most on what happens in that ten- or fifteen-minute encounter between patient and doctor. Patients might get a balanced picture of the benefits and the adverse effects, and a chance to weigh the options. Or they might be sent home with nothing more than an illegible scrawl on a prescription blank. The doctor might recommend the right drug. Or the drug selected could be ineffective, inappropriate, or even dangerous. The purpose of this chapter's visit to offices of the nation's 525,000 doctors is to observe what happens when a drug is prescribed. Sadly, this pivotal link in the safety chain turns out to be one of the weakest.

It should be said at the outset that the world of medicine is populated by many doctors who are bright, well-trained, and conscientious. They put in extra hours to do the best they possibly can for their patients. They stay well informed. This chapter does not pretend to stand in judgment over individual doctors, their efforts on patients' behalf, or the quality of their concern. In a well-engineered system, it is reasonable to expect excellent results from a well-trained professional of average ability. On the other hand, a badly flawed system can make a mockery of the best of intentions. This chapter will examine the scientific evidence about the system, rather than attempt to judge the individual doctors who try to make this system work.

The first peek behind the door into the doctor's office comes at an arthritis clinic affiliated with Harvard Medical School. A researcher named Jeffrey Katz wanted to observe what happened when Harvard's arthritis specialists prescribed a nonsteroidal anti-inflammatory drug such as Oruvail, ibuprofen, naproxen, Orudis, or Feldene.[4] Both patients and doctors consented to having their conversation recorded to study "doctor-patient communication." In particular, Katz wanted to know what these doctors told their patients about the dangers of the drugs they prescribed. With anti-inflammatory drugs, this discussion was not a trivial or technical matter. As seen earlier, the long-term use of anti-inflammatory drugs is so harmful to the stomach and intestinal tract that about 25 percent of the people who take them will seek medical treatment over one year's time. Another 2 to 4 percent will be severely injured.

It is important for doctors to tell patients about these risks for two reasons. The first is patient safety. Patients on long-term anti-inflammatory therapy need to pay special attention to the warning signs of damage to their stomach. The second reason is ethical. The doctor is proposing a medical treatment with substantial, well-documented risks. It is the moral obligation of the doctor to outline both the risks and the benefits of a proposed medical treatment. With an elite medical school faculty involved in Katz's project, we can assume the doctors know the risks of anti-inflammatory drugs. And given a study of "doctor-patient communication," these Harvard doctors ought to be taking care while talking to their patients.

Here are the results: One-quarter of the patients got no information whatever about the adverse effects of the anti-inflammatory drug that was prescribed. Among those who got some information, the main warning was that it might upset their stomach. More than 85 percent of the patients were never warned about the two serious risks of long-term therapy—a perforated ulcer or intestinal bleeding. These findings may surprise the reader, but the principal investigator said at the outset he expected patients would be told little about the dangers of the drugs. As a physician, he knew very well that many doctors do not tell patients about the serious risks of drugs. This fact has been repeatedly confirmed in studies published over decades. For example, in 1994 the FDA conducted a nationwide survey of patients who had recently gotten a prescription from their doctor. More than 70 percent said their doctor told them nothing whatever about the adverse effects of the drugs prescribed.[5] About one-third said they went home without even a doctor's instructions on how much medication to take or when to take it.

Words like "inadequate" or "a major breakdown" do not begin to describe a safety system in which an overwhelming majority of physicians do not meet their ethical obligation of obtaining informed consent to drug therapy, or safeguard their patients by warning them about dangerous adverse effects. Informed consent is a patient right enshrined in the common law since early in this century. It is confirmed by prestigious panels such as the 1982 President's Commission for the Study of Ethical Problems in Medicine. That panel concluded, for example, that a doctor "has an obligation to allow patients to choose from medically acceptable treatment options, or to reject all options."[6] Furthermore, informed consent is not some theoretical right of interest to specialists in medical ethics. In overwhelming numbers, patients and consumers say they want to know all the facts about their health. In one national survey, 96 percent of consumers said they wanted to know possibly the worst of all medical news, a diagnosis of an advanced cancer.[7] Given this preference for harsh reality, it is reasonable to infer that patients would not wish to be shielded from unpleasant news about drug risks.

In another survey, 89 percent of mothers said they wanted to know the exact risk that their child might die from anesthesia, even if the risk was low.[8] In a study of epilepsy medication, from 88 to 98 percent of patients (or parents of children) said they wanted to be informed of various serious risks of the drugs.[9] Ninety-four percent of these patients wanted to be informed of serious but quite rare side effects such as the immune system disorder called lupus. In equally large numbers, they wanted to know about benefits. The epilepsy drug study showed that while patients wanted this information, doctors seldom provided it. As might be expected, doctors were about twice as likely to explain the benefits as the risks.

Why don't doctors give patients this information? Such an overwhelming gap between what is needed and what is provided must have some explanation. In studying the prescription of neuroleptic drugs for severe mental illness, one of the deepest and most disturbing reasons for physician silence may be found. Drugs such as Haldol, Orap, and Thorazine have been greeted as "wonder drugs" that have greatly reduced the populations of mental institutions since the introduction of the first such drugs in the 1950s. Like many drugs, their benefits have been widely advertised while little has been said about their risks. Neuroleptic drugs do not cure mental illness. They do suppress a wide spectrum of behavior, including the voices, delusions, and other manifestations of severe mental illness. As one major drug text explains, "Neuroleptic drugs reduce initiative and interest in the environment, as well as manifestations of emotions or affect."[10] The text declares the effects in humans and animals similar, noting "the animal appears to be indifferent to most stimuli, although it continues to withdraw from those that are noxious or painful. Many learned tasks can still be performed if sufficient stimulation and motivation are provided."[11] Many patients or their legal guardians might accept this diminished capacity as the price paid for relieving the symptoms of severe mental illness. But they certainly ought to explore the risks and benefits with the prescribing physician.

However, as noted in an earlier chapter, the gravest danger of neuroleptic drugs is the damage to the areas of the brain that control voluntary muscle movements. This usually irreversible brain damage, called tardive dyskinesia, appears in 40 percent of patients getting long-term treatment with neuroleptic drugs.[12] It would be hard to think of a stronger case in point to argue that treatment should not begin without a careful discussion of the risks and benefits. Yet of the many dangers of neuroleptic drugs, tardive dyskinesia is the one adverse effect that psychiatrists are least likely to disclose. In one survey of sixty psychiatrists, two-thirds said they did not disclose the risks of tardive dyskinesia to patients. As one doctor explained, "The only thing I have a hard time telling them about is tardive dyskinesia. . . . And the reason I have a hard time is that when I tell them, they will say, 'I don't want to take it.' "[13] Another psychiatrist noted directly, "Specifically, physicians sometimes withhold information about tardive dyskinesia because they believe the patients will refuse to continue taking the medication."[14] There, laid bare, is one reason why doctors don't want to talk about the adverse effects of drugs. They have reached a medical conclusion about what is best for the patient. But given the same facts, the patient or family might reject this advice. The doctor has no ethical or legal right to prevent the patient and family from making an informed decision.

Doctors sometimes gloss over the informed-consent problem by assuming incorrectly that patients don't want to be involved and expect the doctor to decide on the proper treatment. In one landmark survey, 88 percent of doctors believed that patients wanted them to decide what was best. But when asked, only 28 percent of the public said they wanted doctors to make the choices; 72 percent said they wanted to share in medical decision making.[15] Many physicians also object when others draw attention to the drug dangers they themselves may not have described to patients. For example, writer Stephen Fried provided a moving account of his wife's terrible adverse reaction to Floxin, the fluoroquinolone antibiotic.[16] It was published in the *Washington Post Magazine*, and summarized in an earlier chapter. The account triggered a typical angry doctor's reply. "Stephen Fried's article was understandably emotional but regrettably scientifically unbalanced," wrote Eugene Sanders, Jr. "I am deeply concerned that as a result the readership may avoid necessary or even lifesaving treatments with the quinolones or other potent new therapeutic agents."[17] The medical response was similar when the ABC News program *20/20* was preparing a segment describing how drugs for irregular heartbeats can cause cardiac arrest (according to a prominent warning on the drug disclosure label). A Utah cardiologist who had learned of the program wrote, "To present a sensationalistic program that may frighten them could have dire consequences and will undoubtedly complicate their care." It is not merely that most doctors fail to inform patients of the risks of prescription drugs. Many doctors don't want patients to learn about them from any source.

At a deeper level, I believe many physicians simply cannot come to terms with the harm they cause to patients. In the worst case, this can lead to almost unbelievable levels of physician denial. Psychiatrist Peter Breggin noted that the psychiatric profession did not admit the widespread brain damage of tardive dyskinesia until decades after neuroleptic drugs were introduced. "For twenty years the profession simply failed to notice that a large percentage of patients were twitching and writhing from the drugs."[18] Physicians could not come to terms with events occurring right in front of their eyes. Another example of physician denial emerged from my book *Deadly Medicine*. When a major clinical trial produced definitive scientific evidence that drugs given for mild irregular heartbeats were causing lethal cardiac arrest, experts pronounced themselves stunned and surprised by the findings. Yet these same authorities on heart rhythm disorders had seen patients literally drop dead in front of their eyes during the early testing of these drugs, attended emergency meetings where such accounts were discussed, or were hired as drug company consultants to study unexplained patient deaths.[19]

For more than fifteen years, doctors' groups have joined the drug industry in blocking patients from getting accurate information about drug dangers from other sources. This is not a paranoid vision of some secret medical conspiracy, but a description of an open political alliance readily documented in the public record. By the year 1979, the FDA was prepared to take official action to insure that patients learned more about the dangers of drugs prescribed for them. Even at this early date, evidence of doctors' failure to warn their patients was already abundant.[20] The FDA proposed that the known risks of each drug should be clearly and understandably described in a simple document called a "patient package insert." A copy would be included with each prescription. The patient package insert would be a shorter and more understandable version of the drug disclosure label—the highly technical but generally accurate scientific summary provided to doctors.

The patient package insert seemed a straightforward solution to an easily documented problem in the drug safety system. However, it triggered bitter opposition from the pharmaceutical industry and medical groups. The FDA pushed ahead, releasing ten samples so physicians could see that these simple brochures would not be a terrible threat. However, in one of the many probusiness compromises of the early Reagan era, the FDA backed off. Instead, in 1982 it accepted a plan for a voluntary industry program. The pharmaceutical industry would fund a national Council on Patient Information and Education, which would get the job of improving the drug information given to patients. The center collected hundreds of studies about "patient compliance." It held conferences. It published a few brochures about medication safety. But the center focused on getting patients to take their medication, a goal consistent with the center's drug industry funding. It did little to insure that patients received accurate information that would allow them to decide whether or not the risks of a drug were worth it. After ten years, it was evident that the voluntary industry program was a complete failure. In the year 1992, the FDA repeated the patient survey it had conducted in 1982 during the fight over patient package inserts. It concluded, "Researchers found no meaningful change . . . in the percentage of patients whose [doctor] instructed them how much or how often to take their medication." The change in physicians' willingness to discuss adverse reactions was also negligible. In 1992, only 29 percent mentioned any adverse effects, compared to 23 percent in 1982. If you were willing to include information leaflets, the total reached a paltry 35 percent who got some information about adverse effects at the doctor's office. The brief FDA survey, however, didn't address whether the information was adequate, or whether the information was like that in the arthritis study previously cited in which three-quarters of the doctors did discuss adverse effects, but only 15 percent of patients heard about the important dangers of perforated ulcer and intestinal bleeding.

Thus, in 1995 the FDA acted once again, but this time with a more modest proposal called "Medguide." The FDA was willing to give the industry until the year 2000 to distribute voluntarily written information to 75 percent of patients, and until 2006 for all of them. The FDA set broad standards but would not review the exact language in each patient brochure—as it had proposed to do in 1980, and now does with the disclosure labels for doctors.[21] Working behind the scenes, the drug industry sought to block even this modest consumer information effort. Without any discussion or floor debate, the Republican-dominated House of Representatives inserted language into the FDA's annual appropriation bill that blocked any action on the Medguide program. In the United States Senate, only an eleventh-hour effort by

Senator Edward Kennedy prevented a complete debacle. Kennedy won for consumers a compromise of sorts. Rather than proceeding with a federal regulation, the FDA would begin discussions with consumer, medical, and industry groups to develop still another voluntary program. This time, however, the job was not simply turned over to industry. Consumer groups such as the Consumers Union, the Public Citizen Health Research Group, and the Women's Health Network had at least a seat at the table to press for full disclosure of the risks of medication.

As the debate continued over this compromise of a compromise, the attitude of the pharmaceutical industry and organized medicine could be plainly seen. When consumer groups demanded that consumers be explicitly warned of the risks of drugs, the American Medical Association objected. "Such biased information," the AMA said, "may frighten many concerned patients to the point of noncompliance with their medication."[22] Once again, one could see plainly the doctors' fear that many patients would reject drugs if accurately informed of their dangers. The AMA was joined in these objections by the American Academy of Family Physicians and the American College of Obstetricians and Gynecologists.[23] Since doctors couldn't or wouldn't do the job, some consumer groups wanted an increased role for pharmacists in counseling patients about drug dangers. Once again, the AMA objected. The association said, "There is little evidence that retail pharmacists are routinely providing patient counseling services or, in fact, are capable of providing these services."

The trade association of the drug industry, PhRMA, also opposed the mild compromise plan that was being drawn up. "We have been impressed with the number and variety of voluntary private sector programs providing information to patients," PhRMA declared.[24] Given the results of the FDA consumer surveys, the drug companies are likely among the few so easily impressed. The compromise plan, PhRMA complained, "emphasizes not the value that drugs provide and the ability of patient information to increase that value, but rather the hazards that drugs may present." One wonders how the drug industry could be surprised that the consumer information plan focused "on the hazards that drugs may present." That was exactly the information being denied to consumers.

Evidence that the real goal of PhRMA and the AMA was to continue to keep consumers in the dark could be seen in another public position of the two groups. Both objected to the FDA's reviewing the program every two years to monitor progress and check whether the information given to consumers was in fact accurate. "We do not believe that was what Congress had in mind," declared PhRMA. The AMA and its physician organization allies agreed: "Our physician organizations vigorously oppose the creation of any entity or mechanism that implies regulation."[25] Any group that truly wanted a conscientious program to inform consumers would not object to the results being checked. And given the long history of failure, any voluntary program without the FDA systematically evaluating the progress was likely to be still another disappointment.

This vigorous opposition to elementary steps to inform consumers about drug risks was intended to stop what might in fact be a serious threat to the established system. A well-oiled medical machine has been remarkably effective in persuading an ever increasing number of people to take more kinds of prescription drugs for longer and longer periods. As noted above, the physician community and drug industry seem to believe the main reason to give patients information about drugs is to induce them to take medication more regularly, to have more "compliant" patients. When the rights of patients or the demands of safety conflict with the promotion and sale of ever larger numbers of drugs, safety loses. It is a system that maximizes the sale of drugs, not the safety of the public, and those who operate it have not tolerated interference with their priorities.

The second major breakdown in the doctor's office is more basic and was discussed briefly in an earlier chapter: Physicians make dangerous numbers of prescribing mistakes. Even more important than telling patients about the risks of the drugs is selecting a drug with the lowest risks and greatest benefits. A patient may be harmed if the physician selects a drug that is not effective against the patient's medical disorder. Not only is the patient exposed to the risk of a drug that won't work; an effective drug could have helped. A patient may be harmed if the dose is too high, too low, or if a drug interaction is overlooked. A patient may be harmed if the physician selects an addictive drug when a drug without this risk was readily available. A patient may be harmed if the physician is not vigilant enough about the special hazards of some widely used drugs. For example, cortisone and prednisone can trigger a life-threatening hormonal system failure when the drug is abruptly halted.[26] A small overdose of digitalis or Lanoxin can provoke a life-threatening irregular heart rhythm.[27] Failure to monitor the blood levels of Coumadin can result in bleeding or loss of protective effect.[28] Careless use of long-acting benzodiazepine tranquilizers in the elderly can result in hip fractures and other injuries.[29] Lives may be lost because physicians overlook opportunities to prescribe lifesaving medication; the classic example is failure to prescribe beta-blockers for patients who have survived a heart attack. A patient may be harmed if the physician does not monitor the patient carefully enough to discontinue a drug when no longer needed or effective; examples of drugs inappropriately used for extended periods include ulcer medication and narcotics for pain. When a valuable drug is prescribed inappropriately, the results can be tragic, despite the best of intentions.

In Washington, D.C., a doctor named Seymour Greenbaum was examining a young girl named Rose Belle Wade.[30] She had the familiar childhood virus of mumps. Although Greenbaum knew or should have known that penicillin has no effect on viruses, he decided to give her an antibiotic shot. The young girl had an allergic reaction so violent that she died on the examining table right in front of Greenbaum's eyes. Allergic reactions to penicillin occur in about 5 percent of the population.[31] However, the rapid and fatal reaction that Rose experienced is extremely rare, occurring in 1 or 2 out of every 100,000 patients,[32] and this example dates from the 1950s. Are a few tragic deaths merely the price we should be prepared to pay for having a drug so valuable as penicillin? Or did something go wrong in the doctor's office? Since the drug doesn't work against a virus, and since there was a risk of harm but virtually no chance of benefit, one had to ask why penicillin was prescribed in this case. Also, indiscriminate use of antibiotics leads to increasing numbers of drug-resistant infectious agents.

Giving antibiotics for viral diseases is a distressingly common practice. A 1996 study examined a sample of 1,439 Kentucky patients who went to the doctor with one of the viruses that cause the common cold. It found that 60 percent of the patients received an inappropriate prescription for antibiotics.[33] In a scientific literature not known for humor, the medical study was titled, "Do Some Folks Think There Is a Cure for the Common Cold?" The conclusion was more somber. "A majority of persons receiving medical care for the common cold are given prescriptions for an unnecessary antibiotic." The authors estimated that about 15 million Americans got an inappropriate antibiotic prescription every year. In the hospital setting, 50 percent of antibiotic use was deemed inappropriate.[34] So why do doctors prescribe a drug that their medical training showed was ineffective and had some risks of an adverse reaction, and occasionally a very serious one?

"Physicians may feel that the failure to prescribe an antibiotic will result in a dissatisfied patient who will seek care elsewhere," the authors of the common cold study concluded. "Thus, the seemingly benign act of prescribing an antibiotic such as amoxicillin for a cold does little physical harm to the patient and keeps the practice economically viable."[35] If the patients were properly informed, they would learn that antibiotics are inappropriate for viral diseases, and that therefore taking them in this setting has some risks, substantial cost, and no benefits. The only reason doctors can persuade themselves to believe patients "expect" such medication is because the profession has long failed to give these patients accurate information. If it did, the "patients-demand-drugs" excuse would come rapidly to an end.

For almost a decade, Jerry Avorn and Stephen Soumerai at Harvard University systematically studied why doctors so frequently prescribe drugs that are harmful or ineffective. As part of an outreach program to improve prescribing practices, they asked 141 New England doctors their reasons for providing inappropriate or ineffective drugs. The largest number—46 percent—claimed that patients demanded the drugs. Here is what doctors said. "Patient demand was the number one problem in trying to reduce inappropriate prescribing," one Vermont physician told them. Another said he prescribed a "virtually useless" vasodilator for elderly patients "because patients demand them." Two said they felt they had to do something for their patients, even if the scientific data showed they weren't helping. Blaming patients is the oldest alibi in medicine. It is hard to believe many patients would spend their own money for expensive drugs if informed the drugs had no benefits and substantial risks.

About one-quarter of the doctors in Avorn's program conceded the drugs wouldn't work but claimed the prescription "had a positive psychological effect on the patients and their families." A New Hampshire doctor said he "always gives patients drugs with names they don't know" to heighten the mystical effect. "If the patient likes it, it's OK," said another. Decades ago, it might have been acceptable for a doctor to provide a harmless nostrum concocted of mysterious herbs. But to make this use of today's powerful prescription drugs, with their inevitable adverse effects, is indefensible. The remaining doctors in Avorn's study—about one-quarter—simply rejected the scientific evidence and relied "on their clinical experience." In short, about three-quarters of doctors were knowingly giving ineffective prescription drugs to fool or cater to patients, and one-quarter were misinformed about the properties of the drugs.

Virtually every patient population is affected by misprescribed drugs. A Michigan study showed that 12.5 percent of pregnant women were prescribed at least one drug that posed a possible risk to the fetus.[36] In Tennessee, more than 25 percent of young children were inappropriately prescribed tetracycline, an antibiotic that can permanently discolor developing teeth.[37] As noted earlier, in California 15 percent of elderly patients were receiving at least one drug that was ineffective or dangerous in that patient population. Another study of elderly patients focused on the most widely used heart drug—Lanoxin, or digoxin. It found that 47 percent of the prescriptions were for inappropriate indications.[38]

In treating a medical condition as universal and basic as a sore throat, serious deficiencies were found. In one study, 56 percent of doctors were found prescribing antibiotics without first getting a throat culture to check if the infection was susceptible to antibiotic drug treatment or were making some other prescribing error.[39] However, in another project, an HMO wanted to do it right and got the throat cultures first. But because of sloppy follow-up, no prescriptions were provided to 10 percent of patients with positive cultures for strep throat—a case where antibiotic treatment is important and valuable.[40]

Physicians fail to correct prescribing mistakes even when it means that patients are going to die as a result. In the year 1989, the physician community received a major shock when the National Institutes of Health released definitive scientific evidence that doctors were inadvertently killing their patients by attempting to treat mild heart rhythm disturbances with drugs for irregular heartbeats.[41] The release of this data caused a storm of publicity in the news media and medical journals that no practicing physician could possibly have missed. One year later, a survey of cardiologists found that 21 percent had not changed their prescribing practices in new patients.[42] Worse yet, 81 percent of doctors surveyed did not take their patients off these drugs despite scientific evidence they provided no benefits and caused cardiac arrest. More than three-quarters of the heart specialists stopped prescribing the drugs for new patients, but were unwilling to contact patients already on the medication to tell them of the dangers, even when their lives were at stake. Sadly, another study suggests this attitude was not an isolated incident.

In the same period that drugs for irregular heartbeats were proving so lethal, another class of drugs was increasingly proven to save lives among those who survived their first heart attack. The beneficial heart drugs were the beta-blockers, and they repeatedly demonstrated lifesaving properties in this vulnerable patient group. (Those who survive a first heart attack face a 10 to 20 percent risk of death in the next year.) A 1996 study of 5,332 elderly patients in New Jersey showed that only 21 percent of eligible heart attack survivors were prescribed these potentially lifesaving beta-blockers.[43] In some cases, doctors preferred the heavily promoted calcium channel blockers—proven ineffective in this patient population since 1989. Once again, lives were lost because of inappropriate physician prescribing practice. About 10 percent of the heart attack survivors lost their lives unnecessarily because they didn't get beta-blockers.[44] In another example, about 6 percent of the heart attack survivors who got inappropriate drugs for irregular heartbeats suffered a preventable cardiac arrest. If the results of these two studies are true for more than 1 million people who suffer heart attacks each year, then tens of thousands are dying from inappropriate prescribing of these drugs alone.

Sometimes the results of prescription drug studies are so bizarre that it is hard to tell exactly what has gone wrong. Two Columbia University psychiatrists examined the results of a nationwide drug survey focusing on benzodiazepine tranquilizers and sleep aids. These are drugs such as Valium, Halcion, and Xanax. "In nearly half the [cases], the use of benzodiazepines perceived by the patients did not correspond to a labeled or literature-supported unlabeled use," they concluded.[45] The use of benzodiazepines was widespread—about 6.2 percent of the adult population of the United States was taking them. One-third said they took them for anxiety and 9 percent said they were for sleep disorders—the expected uses. However, 15 percent of the patients said they were taking the drugs for high blood pressure or other circulatory problems. Others said the drugs had been prescribed for fungus infections, swelling of the ankles, fluid in the lungs, and anemia. Tranquilizers do not have beneficial effects on these disorders. "Although we cannot rule out the possibility that these examples represent patient-level misperceptions rather than physician-level prescribing practices, closer study is clearly warranted," the authors said.[46] It is a dangerous situation whether the physician failed to tell the patients why they were taking tranquilizers or were prescribing them for the wrong disorders.

At the most critical link in the safety chain—the physician's office—the degree of failure is breathtaking. Three-quarters of patients were not told about the adverse effects of prescribed drugs. Nearly two-thirds of people seeking treatment for the common cold got an ineffective and possibly dangerous prescription for an antibiotic. Eight out of ten heart attack survivors didn't get beta-blockers. One-half of the patients were prescribed the powerful heart drug Lanoxin for inappropriate reasons. One-half of the people prescribed potentially addictive tranquilizers were taking them for purposes for which they could not benefit, or didn't know the purpose of drug treatment. In a responsible system operated with trained professionals, we should be trying to see how far below 1 percent the error rate could be reduced.

Another serious problem in the physician's office is the failure to respond to warnings about newly discovered drug dangers. When the FDA or the drug companies identify a new hazard of drugs, the typical response is some form of warning to doctors. The outright withdrawal of a drug for safety reasons is rare. Among 3,200 drugs on the market, only 14 in the United States were withdrawn for safety reasons from 1970 to 1994, and all but 2 were voluntary withdrawals by the manufacturer. (However, the FDA did pressure the manufacturers to act in some technically voluntary cases.) A warning is a more typical response to a newly discovered drug danger. These are so frequent that every single month there are ten to fifteen drug disclosure label changes—most of them warnings, new adverse effects, or other safety information. When the antihistamine Seldane was linked to cardiac arrests with as little as one extra pill, the initial response was a warning.[47] When the heart drug Tambocor was found to increase the risk of cardiac arrest in heart attack survivors, the response was a warning. When the epilepsy drug Felbatol was found to destroy the bone marrow, the result was a warning. When anti-inflammatory drugs such as ibuprofen and Feldene were discovered to be causing thousands of hospitalizations for perforated ulcers, the response was a warning. When unopposed estrogen was linked to endometrial cancer, the remedial action was a warning. When the painkiller Darvon (and Darvocet-N) was blamed for more than 1,000 overdose deaths every year, the corrective action was a warning to doctors. When the painkiller Zomax was discovered to cause serious allergic reactions, the initial response was a warning. When adverse reaction reports blamed the painkiller Ultram for addiction and seizures, the response was a warning to doctors. As we saw earlier, doctors seldom pass along to patients these warnings—or any other warnings—about adverse effects. Worse yet, the evidence shows that a majority of doctors either don't get or don't respond to warnings.

The main place a new drug warning, adverse effect, or other safety message appears is somewhere in the densely worded drug disclosure label. There is no organized system to make sure doctors see the ten or twenty safety-related changes in drug labels that are made every month. A few disclosure label changes are prominently displayed in boldface type right at the top. More typically they are buried without comment and worded in dense, difficult-to-understand language. Consider the warning for Tambocor, the drug for irregular heartbeats that caused cardiac arrest in about 6 percent of the heart patients who took it for one year. The FDA says this drug should only be used in patients with a life-threatening electrical breakdown of the ventricles. Here is the label warning:

TAMBOCOR was included in the National Heart, Lung and Blood Institute's Cardiac Arrhythmia Suppression Trial (CAST), a long-term, multicenter, randomized, double-blind study in patients with asymptomatic, non-life-threatening ventricular arrhythmias who had a myocardial infarction more than six days but less than two years previously. An excessive mortality or non-fatal cardiac arrest rate was seen in patients treated with Tambocor compared with that seen in a carefully matched placebo-treated group. This rate was 16/315 (5.1%) for Tambocor and 7/309 (2.3%) for its matched placebo. The average duration of treatment with Tambocor in this study was 10 months.[48]

After another 150 words of densely worded text, the warning works toward the punch line:

The applicability of CAST results to other populations (e.g. those without recent infarction) is uncertain, but at present it is prudent to consider the risks of Class IC agents, coupled with the lack of any evidence of improved survival, generally unacceptable in patients whose ventricular arrhythmias are not life-threatening, even if the patients are experiencing unpleasant but not life-threatening symptoms or signs.

It is hard to imagine a more difficult-to-understand warning for already busy physicians. To estimate the severity of the danger, the doctor would have to do the complex arithmetic in his head, subtracting the treatment group from the placebo group and then adjusting the remainder to a standard one-year mortality rate.[49] The key language of the treatment recommendation ("generally unacceptable") was hidden in the middle of another unreadable sixty-five-word sentence. It is hard to blame doctors for failing to heed warnings worded in this manner. In court, the company can claim that it warned doctors (and through these "learned intermediaries," the patients) about the danger of this drug. In fact, it is not an effective warning even though in this instance 3M, the manufacturer, sent doctors similar language in a separate letter.

The scientific record shows that warnings about drug dangers have little effect on doctors' willingness to prescribe drugs. For example, prescriptions for the antibiotic chloramphenicol *rose* after an FDA warning that it could cause lethal destruction of the bone marrow. The manufacturer, Parke-Davis, stepped up its advertising and promotion to keep sales growth on track.[50] There was no effect on prescription volume when a special warning letter was sent to doctors reporting that Zomax frequently caused allergic reactions.[51] And there was only a small effect on prescription volume of Darvon despite a sustained campaign to warn doctors about its addictive properties. Thinking the problem might be hard-to-read warnings that got lost in the mail, Stephen Soumerai and Jerry Avorn of Harvard University tried mailing doctors professionally prepared four-color brochures that were designed to be attention-getting and easy to read. The information was identified as coming from the Harvard Medical School Drug Information Program. The mailed brochures alone had no effect in reducing inappropriate prescribing by doctors.[52] Soumerai and Avorn found that prescribing patterns changed only when such information was accompanied by face-to-face contact in an office visit or drug symposium.

The widespread failure of physicians to respond to FDA and manufacturers' warnings about drug dangers renders the basic system ineffective. Consider the risks of Halcion, which were explored in chapter 9. Rather than withdrawing the drug (as was done in Britain), one FDA response was a strong warning to doctors not to prescribe Halcion for more than 7 to 10 days. However, the 1996 report of the FDA's Halcion Task

Force concluded that despite the warning, 85 percent of prescriptions were for longer than the recommended period.

So what are we to do about physician prescribing mistakes? Decades of experience in the business of quality control has shown that punishment, blame, and criticism probably will have little effect. When few patients ever find out that they were the victim of prescribing error, there is little or no incentive for doctors to change. There is no government, public or nonprofit agency, panel, board, foundation, or other entity charged with improving doctors' prescribing practices. Finally, without collecting more systematic information about prescribing errors, it is hard to know exactly where to start. So how does this change?

First, we need better-informed and more vigilant consumers, with a better chance of getting prescribing errors fixed. Later chapters in this book will explain what consumers can do. Physicians are sensitive to what they hear from patients. Second, while few people in this era would suggest that the federal government ought to regulate doctors' prescribing practices, it should collect information about the most dangerous and common problems. The federal government already collects health information about illness, smoking, vaccinations, auto accidents, causes of death, and a host of other issues. In order to make progress, we need better information about inappropriate prescribing. Next, doctors need better computer tools to help them prescribe drugs more wisely. Even though physicians may deal with five hundred to a thousand different drugs in daily medical practice, they are still trained to prescribe drugs purely from memory. (When was the last time you saw a doctor consult a drug reference before prescribing a drug for you?) One reason why doctors tell patients so little about the adverse effects of drugs is that they can't possibly remember all of them. One reason they fail to heed warnings is that they never receive them. Finally, the growing revolution in managed care may offer new opportunities to improve drug safety. About one-third of prescriptions now flow through pharmacy benefit manager organizations for approval. The same system designed to encourage doctors to use cheaper drugs could help doctors prescribe safer drugs. Nevertheless, the system will respond best to a concerned public. Little will change until alarmed consumers realize they have about a 1-in-5 chance of getting an inappropriate or dangerous drug, and demand something better than this dismal result.

CHAPTER ELEVEN

Fixing the System

IN THE SPRING and summer of 1996, groups of concerned citizens traveled to Washington, D.C., to seek major changes in the way the FDA reviews and approves new drugs. They came from Overland Park, Kansas, and North Freedom, Wisconsin; from Southfield, Michigan, and Marshalltown, Iowa. They were not doctors or pharmacologists, just citizens from Main Street, USA. After arriving in Washington, they wanted to talk to their senators and representatives about reforming the FDA. Voters who visit Washington with political change on their minds have a more powerful voice than one might suppose in a town known to cater to celebrity television reporters and power lobbyists. The delegation easily got appointments to voice their concerns; some met personally with a member of Congress while others saw the legislative assistant who handled FDA matters.

These citizens were not concerned about the safety issues that have been the focus of this book. In fact, they were urging members of Congress to curb the powers of the FDA and reduce the requirements for drug testing, believing this would help them get powerful new medicines quickly. They had heartbreaking stories to tell. One had a beloved spouse who was being slowly paralyzed by multiple sclerosis. Another told of her child who could experience a hundred seizures a day. A woman who helped other women cope with life after breast cancer surgery had seen the need for better drugs with her own eyes, every day. They were desperate for any medicine to help. Their plight was made more difficult, they believed, by the FDA's elaborate requirements for drug testing. At first glance, this looks like American democracy as it is supposed to work. Almost every week elected officials were hearing from one or more of their constituents who were critical of the FDA and wanted action taken. They were well informed about the issues. This seemed to be evidence of a groundswell of public concern of the kind that truly does create change.

In fact, something quite different than it appeared was taking place. Hardly anyone is more vulnerable than the victim of a slowly advancing but lethal illness, or the parent of a child who is seriously ill. The pharmaceutical industry was executing a carefully conceived plan to exploit these vulnerable people for political gain. PhRMA, the industry association, sensing the probusiness leanings of the first Republican majority in Congress in decades, had launched an ambitious plan to rewrite the laws that govern drug safety and testing. Drug testing and research is a major industry expense, second only to marketing and advertising.[1] Reducing drug testing, and therefore industry costs, was a seemingly sure route to increased profits. The concerned citizens were just another element in a coordinated campaign that featured professional lobbyists, television advertising, letters from health groups, and symposia for congressional members and staff. The pseudopopulist tone of this initiative engineered by the most profitable business in the world could be seen in the industry newsletter. It was called *The Patient Advocate*.

The pharmaceutical industry had gone to much trouble and considerable expense to create the illusion of public support for lowering drug safety standards. Earlier in the year, PhRMA had hired consultants in local communities across the country. Their job was to find families in which someone was severely ill and possibly concerned about drugs. Then the targets were interviewed by telephone to see if they sounded agreeable to the industry position. The suitable candidates were flown to Washington at industry expense. Their hotel bills, meals, and other expenses were also paid. A PhRMA representative often escorted the groups right to the door of a representative's office before disappearing from sight. This scheme came to the attention of John Schwartz, a reporter for the *Washington Post*. He told PhRMA he wanted to talk to patients whose problems would be solved by the industry's plan to curb the FDA.

When Schwartz checked into these patients' problems, he discovered the FDA was not to blame for their problems.[2] For example, Janet McDermott of Marshfield, Massachusetts, complained that an epilepsy medication she needed for her daughter was available in Canada but not in the United States. The delay, Schwartz learned, was mainly caused by the drug company, Hoechst Marion Roussel. It had been slow in submitting the required information to the FDA. Stephanie Hudson of St. Louis complained that the drug used to treat her child's sickle-cell anemia was not FDA-approved to treat this particular medical condition. While the drug was available, it was still hard to get insurance companies to pay for treatment. However, Schwartz found the manufacturer,

Bristol-Myers Squibb, had never sought FDA approval for this medical use.

The industry's efforts to rewrite the drug safety laws failed in the election-year Congress, in large part because the industry's claim to represent patients angered and mobilized the genuine grassroots consumer organizations. However, with so much money at stake, the industry will undoubtedly continue to press for changes that will benefit it. The industry drive to lower drug-testing standards and reduce the FDA's authority make a fitting backdrop for this chapter. They dramatize the truth that change can and does occur all the time. The industry did have one part right. It understood that change occurs when informed and concerned citizens insist that their elected representatives take action. Much can be accomplished to reduce the toll of severe injury and death from prescription drugs.

Change for the better must begin with better information about drug safety. It would be hard to imagine the Federal Aviation Administration trying to improve airline safety without knowing whether any airplanes had crashed in the last year. Could a police chief create a safer community without knowing how many crimes occurred, or how many arrests? How effective could the nation's programs to insure the safety of nuclear power reactors be with no accurate information about their operating problems? Could we build cars that are safer to drive without accident data? Yet the FDA has the job of protecting the public from the dangers of drugs without knowing how many people are getting hurt. No one knows whether deaths and serious injuries are increasing, stable, or rapidly declining. We cannot single out the most dangerous drugs for added special precautions.

Here is a sample of the 1994 results from the FDA's existing Spontaneous Reporting System.[3] Let's see what can be learned about the safety of drugs from this data.

RANK	DRUG	MEDICAL USE[4]	CASES
1	Prozac	depression	2,055
2	Risperdal	anti-psychotic	1,777
3	Clozaril	anti-psychotic	1,554
4	Paxil	depression	1,315
5	Proscar	enlarged prostate	1,238

Two drugs for depression—Prozac and Paxil—caused more reported adverse reactions than any drug to treat cancer, prevent seizures, combat pain, control diabetes, cure infections, or prevent pregnancy. Does this signal a safety problem? Or does it merely reflect the popularity and successful marketing of drugs for depression? It is hard to tell because the data are not good enough. Even crude sales data don't help much. Prozac was the no. 10 best-seller in 1994, but ranked first in adverse reactions. Is Paxil safer than Prozac, or more dangerous? Paxil trailed far behind Prozac in 1994 in sales, ranking no. 59.[5] Because adverse reactions ranked higher than sales, we might wonder whether Paxil is more dangerous. By 1996, Paxil increased its market share. Were more people being sold a drug with a higher chance of causing them harm? We don't know for sure. But a good system with reliable findings could steer patients toward the safest alternative. These are some of the questions that could be answered if we had better, more reliable information about drug safety.

How concerned should we be about the grand total of 2,055 reported adverse reactions for Prozac? In a given year, Prozac is taken by hundreds of thousands of people. Since so many people take the drug, a total of 2,055 reports could be interpreted as evidence the drug is pretty safe. Because the reporting is voluntary, we have no idea whether 1 out of every 100, or even 1 out of 1,000 adverse reactions, was reported. Consider what the FDA learned about the heart drug Lanoxin. It is even more widely used than Prozac, ranking no. 9 on the 1994 list of best-sellers. The FDA adverse reaction reports suggest that Lanoxin is causing few problems despite being given to older people with ailing and injured hearts. From 1985 to 1992, the FDA received an average of 82 spontaneous reports a year of adverse reactions to Lanoxin.[6] It would appear that there is nothing much to worry about. Researchers decided to check the computerized hospital records for the Medicare program. In the same seven-year period, they identified 202,011 cases where the adverse effects of Lanoxin were so severe they required hospitalization.[7] The authors warned that their computer study probably failed to identify many cases. In the case of Lanoxin, the FDA system captured only 1 out of every 362 serious cases. If the same proportions were true for Prozac, it could be causing more than 700,000 adverse reactions in a single year. Unfortunately, we really can't tell whether doctors and nurses are more likely to report an adverse reaction to Prozac than a problem with Lanoxin.

The truth is we don't know what's happening. Voluntary, spontaneous reports rarely provide information that is reliable enough to justify corrective action. As a first step toward improving drug safety, we need to build a better information system to identify the most important drug dangers reliably. Another approach might be to instruct the experts at the FDA to investigate further these early indications that a drug safety problem might exist. The tiny FDA division that is responsible for monitoring the safety of approved drugs has eight professionals trained as doctors or epidemiologists and assigned to investigate such questions.[8] With 3,200 approved drugs in daily use, this is grossly inadequate. The Nuclear Regulatory Commission employs more than 1,000 professionals to monitor 109 reactors; the FAA deploys 10,000 trained inspectors for about 5,000 commercial airliners. The far greater danger of drugs has a safety monitoring staff totaling 54 people.

The first step toward safer drugs is crucial and relatively inexpensive. We have to find out how many people are now being injured by drugs, and why. To do this requires a much larger staff of specialists trained to investigate safety issues. They need adverse reaction reporting systems that don't depend on the chance that a doctor or a nurse might report a drug reaction. They need the power and the money to do follow-up studies, and new tools to take action against drug dangers. I have described elsewhere my own ideas in greater detail.[9] A campaign to improve drug safety will achieve very little without accurate and regular reporting to identify the biggest dangers and monitor our progress toward overcoming them. Solving the next major safety problem will cost more.

Except for one giant loophole, the testing and FDA evaluation of new drugs is one of the stronger links in the system. The clinical trials that must prove a drug is effective are so rigorous that 50 percent of the drugs that enter human testing fail.[10] The FDA closely monitors the testing; its medical and statistical specialists are widely respected for their expertise. The approval of new drugs is such a high priority at the FDA that it commands about 75 percent of the staff time and budget for drug regulation. (By comparison, the surveillance and monitoring of approved drugs gets less than 5 percent.) Despite the healthy rigor of the FDA scrutiny before drug approval, a major loophole has opened our society to risks so great they are difficult to imagine.

While the evaluation of new drugs is rigorous, the testing periods are also short, often a matter of a few weeks, or a few months. For an antibiotic taken for ten days to cure strep throat, a short trial seems reasonable. But what about the many drugs that must be taken for months or years to maintain their effect? People take for the rest of their lives drugs to lower blood pressure and cholesterol, to maintain thyroid hormone levels, and to replace estrogen. Drugs for depression or other mental illness can be prescribed for many years. These drugs are also tested for very short periods of time. Consider a new and best-selling drug for more severe mental illness, Risperdal. Here is what the manufacturer reports:

> The antipsychotic efficacy of RISPERDAL® was established in short-term (6 to 8 weeks) controlled trials of schizophrenic in-patients. The effectiveness of RISPERDAL® in long-term use, that is, more than 6 to 8 weeks, has not been systematically evaluated in controlled trials. Therefore, the physician who elects to use RISPERDAL® for extended periods should periodically re-evaluate the long-term usefulness of the drug for the individual patient.[11]

You don't have to be a psychiatrist to know that these drugs don't cure mental illness—they only suppress the most extreme behavior, and along with it desirable behavior. While they may be used for brief periods in psychiatric wards to contain a psychotic crisis, a more typical use is for years on end. Yet, Risperdal was approved without knowing anything about its long-term effects—good or bad.

On the other hand, it doesn't make sense to require multimillion-dollar drug testing just to keep the research documentation tidy. Are there credible reasons to suppose that long-term use of Risperdal might be hazardous? In this case, the answer is yes. The American Psychiatric Association, as noted earlier, reported that brain damage occurs in about 40 percent of the patients who took similar drugs over the long term.[12] If Risperdal causes less brain damage than Haldol or other established drugs, then it may be a godsend. But what if Risperdal produces beneficial changes in behavior in the short run, but even greater damage to the brain with continued use?

Without systematic long-term testing, we'll never know. In the meantime, all we have is the reports in the table above that show Risperdal triggered more adverse reaction reports than any other drug except Prozac. Similar questions about long-term effects remain unanswered concerning drugs to combat depression. The clinical trials for Prozac, Paxil, Zoloft, and Effexor lasted only five to six weeks, even though months to years of therapy are common.[13]

Consider the case of Ritalin, examined in the opening chapter. It is being taken by millions of young children for its short-term effects on behavior. Long-term effects are unknown. Ritalin is a drug that proved dangerous in animal testing, causing cancer and changes in brain chemistry. Ritalin has proved addictive in adults. Are we supposed to believe—without scientific evidence—that Ritalin is perfectly safe when used by children over the long term? Are they somehow exempt from the harm we observed in animal testing and college students and adults? And are we so confident of that proposition that we do not want to insist on long-term testing? Nowhere in the law or in FDA policy is such long-term testing required. Even though Ritalin has been a profitable drug for decades, no such studies have been performed.

Two cholesterol-lowering drugs, Atromid-S and Pravachol, illustrate another dimension to long-term testing. In short-term tests, both drugs reduced cholesterol levels. Many people would accept the theory that since higher cholesterol signals a higher risk of heart attack, then lowering blood cholesterol ought to be beneficial. Such drugs are typically taken for a lifetime. Is there a good reason to want long-term testing? Again, the answer is yes, but for a different reason. The true health benefits—a lower risk of heart attack—occur only over the long term. No one, even the patient, could observe any immediate effects of either Pravachol or Atromid-S. If either drug has a tangible health effect, it would occur over the long term.

While the long-term effects of most drugs remain unknown, these two were tested. Long-term testing revealed that Pravachol saved lives and prevented heart attacks.[14] It performed as well as, and possibly better than, researchers had hoped. However, long-term testing of Atromid-S revealed that it increased the risk of dying rather than reducing it.[15] In a long-term trial sponsored by the World Health Organization, the death rate was 25 percent higher among those taking the active drug, compared to patients taking an inactive placebo.[16] In this rare case where long-term testing was performed, it revealed a world of difference between two drugs that both lowered cholesterol. One was beneficial and saved lives. The other increased the death rate in a well-conducted clinical trial. But in short-term testing, both appeared to be effective in lowering cholesterol.

Thus, we need long-term testing to detect risks that may emerge only with several years of use. We also need long-term testing to check whether the expected benefits in fact exist. In a third example, the FDA, doctors, and patients have accepted a family of drugs for thirty years despite evidence the drugs may be harmful when taken over the long term. Today hundreds of thousands of Americans take drugs such as Glucotrol, Micronase, or DiaBeta to reduce mild elevations of blood sugar. It is a case somewhat similar to cholesterol. Particularly in people who are obese, laboratory tests frequently reveal mild elevations of blood sugar, a condition now called Type 2 diabetes. Most have no symptoms. The drugs have been proven effective in the short term in reducing blood sugar levels. But does reducing blood sugar produce health benefits or prevent harmful complications over the long term? If it does not, then treatment is at best pointless and more likely, dangerous. A clinical trial was launched to answer that question, taking nearly a decade to complete. The results shocked the diabetes specialists who had long advocated drug treatment.

Treatment with one key drug not only had no health benefits, it more than doubled the risk of death from heart disease—already the top health hazard of Type 2 diabetes.[17] Some patients with type 2 diabetes are also treated with insulin. The study showed no benefits of this treatment, but no suggestion of harm either. One might imagine that with uncontradicted scientific evidence that drug treatment of Type 2 diabetes was harmful, and insulin treatment of no benefit, that doctors would take patients off these drugs. But that is not what happened. The American Diabetes Association declared, "Careful evaluation of the complete data and further study will be necessary. At this point the evidence available does not warrant abandoning any of the presently accepted methods of treatment of diabetes."[18] Since about 95 percent of the people said to have "diabetes" have only these mild elevations of blood sugar, calling a halt to treatment would have threatened the future of the entire medical specialty.

With an important warning flag now clearly in view, one would suppose "the further study" would be promptly undertaken, and clear evidence of long-term benefits established in clinical trials. In 1997, the American Diabetes Association proposed a massive new health initiative to test every adult in the United States over forty-five in order to identify and treat millions more people with smaller elevations of blood sugar than are currently treated, people with no overt symptoms of ill health.[19] In this classic rush to treatment, only a few words of caution could be heard. David Nathan, a Harvard University diabetes specialist, told the *New York Times*: "We start with diet and exercise and rather rapidly move into a number of drugs without data to suggest that's good for patients over a long time. We must be careful we don't cause some mischief, don't make their heart disease worse."[20] The original study showing that at least one of these agents appeared to be harmful was completed in 1970. Twenty-seven years later the long-

:erm benefits—or even safety—of drug treatment of Type 2 diabetes have yet to be established.

Millions of Americans today might be taking drugs that are slowly poisoning them rather than providing a health benefit because of the systemwide failure to insist on long-term drug testing. Seven million people take calcium channel blockers—drugs such as Procardia, Norvasc, Cardizem, and Calan—for mild elevations of blood pressure. Because of failure to do long-term testing, no one can say whether they are beneficial, harmful, or ineffective in reducing the health risks of hypertension. Tens of thousands of people with cancer take highly toxic drugs that are proven to reduce the size of tumors. Many of these drugs were never tested to determine whether over the long term the toxic side effects outweigh the medical benefits—either in quality of life or increased survival.

Why, then, has such a large gap been permitted in society's defenses against the dangers of drugs? First, because both doctors and patients are willing to embrace unproven new drugs. In such a marketplace, why would drug companies pay for expensive testing to document the true benefits of their drugs when doctors will accept a vastly cheaper mix of optimism and untested medical theory? When market mechanisms fail—and the market rarely works well on issues of safety—the alternative is for society to insist on such testing as a matter of law. However, if long-term testing were a precondition for initial approval, it might introduce prohibitive delays. Instead of taking ten years to bring a drug to market, it might take fifteen years for drugs that required long-term testing. Testing is especially lengthy when the benefits of the drug are so small that it takes observing thousands of patients to measure a small effect. For example, Merck had to study 4,444 patients for up to 6.3 years to document that its cholesterol drug Zocor had prevented seventy-eight serious coronary events.[21] While costs are high, so are the rewards. Zocor might have cost $30 million or more to test. But in 1996, Zocor produced more than $1 billion in revenue for Merck.[22] The necessary long-term testing of drugs could be assured through several kinds of mechanisms. The long-term testing could be performed as a public or private enterprise. It could be paid for with tax dollars, with a 1 percent tax on drugs that required such testing, or with a tax levied directly on the companies that market these highly profitable products. However, it ought to be unacceptable to spend billions of dollars every year on long-term drug treatment without knowing whether it is beneficial, or whether people are unwittingly paying hard-earned money to harm their own health.

The failure to monitor injuries and deaths and the lack of long-term drug testing are the two most serious faults in the system. The third major problem, the focus of the previous chapter, is prescribing errors by doctors. It is ironic that society has taken away from consumers the right to select their own drugs—and control their own bodies—because drugs are so powerful and risky it requires an expert or learned intermediary. Yet when the performance of these experts is examined, error rates of 15 percent, 20 percent, and even 50 percent of prescriptions written were found. In any reasonably managed safety system, the question ought to be how far below 1 percent the error rate can be reduced. Part of the solution to this serious problem is straight-forward, part very difficult. The route to reducing errors in complex tasks has been described in literally hundreds of books about quality control. Consensus exists about what works. It doesn't help to blame the person who makes the error—the problem usually is a system that needs to be improved. The results have to be measured and analyzed continuously so the people in the system know what they are doing right and wrong, and can see their progress. We need to develop tools that minimize the chances for errors. Every time I see a doctor scrawl a prescription in handwriting, relying entirely on memorized information, I see an accident waiting to happen. Did the doctor remember the warning letter that came two weeks ago in a large stack of mail? How could he know about the drug another specialist prescribed for me? The traditional use of easily confused abbreviations such as b.i.d.(twice a day) and q.i.d. (four times a day) is an invitation to error because the difference between a *b* and a *q* may depend on a small squiggle of handwriting. More alarming yet are hospital error studies showing that lethal drug accidents are frequently caused by a tenfold error—omitting or misplacing a decimal point and thus possibly ordering a 1 mg dose instead of a .1 mg dose.)[23]

We need to reengineer the doctor's office. There are no losers here. Everyone would benefit. Patients would be safer. Doctors could use their time more effectively to help sick people get better. Expensive injuries and hospitalizations would be prevented. This is the easy part. The hard part has to do with how modern medicine is organized.

There is no mandate for change. Consumers rarely know when they are victims of prescribing errors. Even when they do learn of a medical mistake, they rarely blame the doctor—unless the error was very serious.[24] The medical literature provides compelling evidence of prescription error, but apparently most doctors think someone else must be making all those mistakes. (This is one reason why monitoring the results is the key to eliminating errors. A doctor who erroneously believes he is making few prescription errors will quickly learn otherwise.) It is a sad testimony to the priorities in medicine today that several nationwide business ventures have been launched to give doctors a fancy computer or interactive television system to present drug company advertising.[25] But there has been no comparable investment in computer-based tools to enhance drug safety. The best hope for progress comes through the profound change that is now transforming the landscape of American medicine. For decades—if not centuries—doctors were solo practitioners or worked with a few colleagues in group practices. Except for malpractice, a doctor's medical judgment reigned supreme. In just a few years, the managed care revolution has ended physician independence. For more than 100 million Americans, when a doctor writes a prescription, it is reviewed by a managed-care organization. (This is one purpose of the prescription benefits cards.) At present, managed care is mainly trying to reduce the cost of the drugs prescribed, substituting a cheaper chemical or therapeutic equivalent. However, the large managed care companies and pharmacy benefit managers that are already monitoring the prescribing practices of doctors present a structure and opportunity to reduce prescription error. Whether managed care companies will see drug safety as another potential benefit—or will narrowly pursue profits and lower costs—remains to be seen.

The three priorities described above—better monitoring, long-term testing, and reduced prescription errors—are the most urgent needs. There is much else to be done. Consumers should have the legal right to the same information about drug dangers that is now given to doctors. Drugs should be rated for toxicity, so patients and doctors can quickly grasp the risks involved. FDA drug approvals should not be permanent. Drugs should be reevaluated every five years in light of postmarketing experience and availability of safer alternatives. Drugs that were the safest of their kind in 1985 might be unacceptably toxic today compared to newer drugs. We need independent centers for research on new ways to improve drug safety and to provide education in using established tools that work. The nation's pharmacists need to study dispensing errors and find a way to more consistently warn consumers about drug interactions. New rules are needed to prevent drug companies from burying warnings about safety in an avalanche of new drug advertising. Consumers should have the prescription drug equivalent of the second opinion on surgery; patients with medication problems need access to an independent evaluation. The federal government is already in the business of promoting wider use of medication—notably blood pressure and cholesterol drugs. Such programs should be balanced with educational campaigns to curb overmedication and inappropriate prescribing. When drug treatment is needed, programs should encourage wider use of the safest and most cost-effective instead of the most aggressively marketed drug in each family. The most common sources of severe injury and death should be attacked on a drug-by-drug basis. Among the urgent problems: perforated ulcers and bleeding from anti-inflammatory drugs; brain damage from antipsychotic drugs; manic attacks from antidepressants; addiction to painkillers; dose errors for Coumadin; use of estrogen without progesterone to prevent endometrial cancer; heart rhythm disruptions from Lanoxin; inadequate monitoring of drugs that destroy bone marrow; harmful use of sedatives and antipsychotics in nursing homes; and cardiac arrest from drugs for irregular heartbeats. The list could continue indefinitely. To accomplish everything recommended in this chapter would consume only a fraction of the $1.5 billion a year that the drug companies spend to persuade doctors to favor their particular drugs.

So what does the drug industry say about safety? A position paper on drug safety from PhRMA provides an example. "Because drugs are powerful substances, they cannot be made completely safe for all users under all circumstances," it notes.[26] This argument is, "We just have to accept a few injuries to get the benefits." Can you imagine the airline industry arguing that having 1 million people seriously injured in airplane crashes every year was just part of the game because air travel can't be "made completely safe for all users under all

circumstances"? Next, the industry blames the patients. "Failure to take medications properly costs more than $100 billion
a year due to increased hospital admissions, nursing home
admissions, lost productivity and premature deaths."[27] Finally, those who do worry about safety just have a distorted
perspective. Notes PhRMA, "There is more attention paid to
rare problems with drugs than to their much more prevalent
benefits." In short, we wouldn't have to be so worried about
drug safety if we would just stop thinking about it. This is like
suggesting that those concerned about auto accident deaths
would be less worried if they just spent more time thinking
about the millions of people who reach their destination safely
every day. Have the pharmaceutical industry and doctors
through their vigilance already taken deaths and serious injuries to some irreducible minimum? To answer that question
we need only turn to the scientific record.

In 1997, David Classen studied adverse drug reactions occurring in 2,227 Salt lake City hospital patients.[28] He judged
that 50 percent of the injuries were preventable. In 1995,
David Bates identified 247 adverse drug reactions at two
Boston area hospitals.[29] Overall, 29 percent were preventable.
In 1992, C. M. Lindley studied 113 elderly patients hospitalized for adverse drug reactions.[30] He found half of all adverse
reactions were caused by drugs administered despite a specific
warning against them or that were unnecessary. In 1991, Susanna Bedell studied cardiac arrests caused by medical treatment in a Boston teaching hospital; 15 of 203 episodes were
caused by preventable medication errors.[31] In 1991, Lucian
Leape and 11 Harvard colleagues studied adverse events of all
types in New York State hospitals.[32] Drug complications were
the single most common adverse event. An expert panel concluded that 17.7 percent of the drug complications were due
to outright negligence. In 1987, Judyann Bigby examined 686
patients in a primary care medical practice who required

emergency hospital admission.[33] Bigby found that 72 percent of the preventable hospitalizations involved prescription drugs. In 1977, Jane Porter examined deaths from adverse drug reactions in a group of Boston area patients. She reported that 25 percent of the deaths might have been preventable.[34] In 1976, John Burnham reviewed all of the adverse drug reactions occurring in his own medical practice. He reported that "55% were unjustifiable and preventable."[35] In 1967, William Best examined 288 cases in which the antibiotic chloramphenicol destroyed the bone marrow, often with lethal effect. The incidence of this adverse effect is extremely rare, occurring in less than 1 in 30,000 cases.[36] It is just the kind of example that leads some to conclude that rare adverse effects are an inescapable cost of having powerful drugs. However, Best found that 75 percent of the victims never should have been given any antibiotic in the first place. The drug was being used for the common cold, acne, and other ailments for which it was not effective. For thirty years, those who have examined the evidence carefully have reached a similar conclusion. They have found that a large fraction of deaths or serious injuries could have been prevented. We know how to do it. We can achieve a better system and a safer system when the public starts to insist. The solutions lie not in vast expenditures of money, or trying to get people to give up drugs they deem beneficial. The solutions lie in basic, prudent steps to minimize the great risks of drugs while still making good use of their substantial benefits.

For many months, I have pondered the stark contrast between the decades-long neglect of drug safety and the intense public concern and vigorous actions taken on other safety issues. In terms of lives at risk, it would be hard to find a more serious problem. As shown earlier, prescription drugs cause 100,000 deaths every year, 1 million injuries so severe they require hospitalization, and another 2 million injuries occurring during hospital care. To combat this risk, the FDA has about 1,600 full-time employees in drug regulation, most of whom focus on new drug applications. Now consider the vigor of the government response to a sensational event that triggers immediate public concern. When 168 people were killed in a terrorist attack on a federal office building in Oklahoma City, the federal government responded by spending $200 million and hiring more than 1,500 new employees to upgrade federal building security. When 241 people were killed in the crash of a TWA flight to Paris, the government spent more than $15 million in an unsuccessful effort to identify the cause of this single crash. The investigation of this one episode cost three times more than the total spent for all safety and monitoring of approved drugs for an entire year. Nevertheless, when safety was at issue, the government was ready to spare no expense. Months after it was clear no proof of terrorist activity could be found—and no group claimed credit—President Clinton announced a massive federal program to combat the threat—whether real or perceived. He announced that fifty-four special bomb detection machines would be installed in airports at a cost of more than $1 million each. The FAA would hire 300 new special agents to add to the 10,000 FAA employees already monitoring the safety of the air system. The FBI would add an additional 644 agents, and these agents would require 620 assistants and other support personnel.

One might be tempted to say that these are political responses to intense fear in the public mind rather than a reasoned response to a measured threat. Yet many examples can be found of vast national safety programs targeted at problems that are nowhere near so dramatic, nor so traumatically embedded in the public psyche as these two episodes. For example, a laudable public health crusade has been launched to persuade bicycle riders to wear helmets to prevent head injuries should they get hit by a car.[37] If every one of the 200 million people who might ride a bicycle would wear a helmet, then about 400 lives a year might be saved.[38] (This would also prevent a much larger number of minor head injuries.) Benefits on a similar scale were hoped for in the national campaign to reduce auto accident deaths. By law, two air bags must be installed in every new motor vehicle at a cost of approximately $300. The safety experts who wanted these measures said they hoped about 300 lives a year might be saved. Compare these laudable programs with the lifesaving potential of an initiative to improve the safety of drugs. Given the estimates of preventable drug events, then an effective drug safety program could save in about three days as many lives as the bicycle and air bag initiatives hope to achieve in one year.

Knee-jerk responses, whether denial or overreaction, seldom save lives in the real world of accident prevention. A rational and measured response is essential. Such a response should begin with much better information about how many people are now being injured and why. Prevention programs should be launched against explicit targets to achieve results that can be objectively measured. It shouldn't be more difficult to help physicians make fewer prescribing errors and persuade consumers to be more alert than to get 35 million children to wear their bicycle helmets.

PART THREE

WHAT YOU CAN DO

CHAPTER TWELVE

The Skeptical Consumer

DRUG SAFETY BEGINS with a sensible attitude. Something buried deep in the ancient ritual of taking medicine seems to provoke the unhealthy extremes—either an unquestioning faith in medication, or an unreasoning fear of harm. Any readers with a blind faith in drugs probably put this book down long ago. But there is less to protect the skeptical consumer from the other extreme—fear that stops people from taking acceptable risks to obtain valuable drug benefits. This hazard was driven home by a friend. We had lunch regularly, and he would often hear one of the stories about the drugs that I was researching. One day, he listened to the vivid story about the corporate lawyer who had been hospitalized with a perforated ulcer after taking the anti-inflammatory drug Oruvail. Later I noticed that my friend was limping badly, and asked what was the matter. He recently had had arthroscopic surgery. After the procedure, his knee had become so swollen that he could hardly move it. I asked which anti-inflammatory drug he was taking. He said the surgeon had prescribed one, but after hearing all the stories about perforated ulcers and other complications, he had not taken the medication. Sorry, but this is the wrong attitude. Inhibiting the body's response to tissue injury after surgery is an example of a case when benefits are likely to outweigh the risks.

Another pain story has a different message. One day I was looking over the medication being taken by an older woman with arthritis. She was taking several different drugs for pain, the most powerful being Vicodin—a combination of a narcotic and acetaminophen. I asked why she was taking it. One year earlier, she had experienced a sudden flare-up of pain in her knee just before leaving on a long-scheduled trip abroad. Vicodin had been prescribed for that emergency. Had the knee problem persisted? Actually, the knee had been just fine for months. After I questioned the need for the drug and she consulted with her doctor, she discontinued the Vicodin without incident. For months, she had been taking—and possibly developing tolerance to—a potentially addictive pain medication which she didn't need at all. Taking powerful prescription drugs is a serious business with genuine risks. The goal is to get the most benefit with the least risk. Thus, the first step toward drug safety is approaching the subject with the right attitude.

The right attitude is that you are the boss—but follow the instructions. A prescription drug changes the settings on the most important control switches in the world—those that operate your own body. As we have seen, even the most familiar drugs, such as aspirin, Seldane, and Tagamet, have profound biological effects. The doctor may select and prescribe the drug. But it is your body and your decision whether the benefits outweigh the risks. The notable exception is a medical emergency or hospital crisis where the need for rapid intervention makes it reasonable to rely heavily on the treating physician. But for most of the drugs a majority of us take most of the time, you're the boss. If there are benefits, you and only you will receive them. If there is harm, you're going to experience it. But given a powerful tool to control the biological operations of your own body, you still need to follow instructions.

If you have enough cash, you can buy a quite different powerful tool—a little corporate jet airplane for your personal use. You'll definitely be the boss; it will take you just about anywhere in the world whenever you want to go. But even though you're the boss, you'd better follow the manufacturer's instructions—for example, landing it at the recommended speed, maintaining it just as the manufacturer suggests. Drugs work in a human machine more complicated than a jet aircraft. You have to follow the instructions. In some people, beta-blockers cause severe enough depression that a heart patient might reasonably decide the harm outweighs the benefit. That's your decision. But the manufacturer's instructions also warn about the dangers of discontinuing beta-blockers abruptly. Quitting this drug is not a do-it-yourself project; you need to see a doctor.

On the other hand, just because you have a heart condition and your doctor prescribed it, you don't have to take this drug no matter how miserable it makes you feel. It's your body. You're the boss—ethically and legally—not the doctor. That said, understand that quitting some drugs requires medical management—such as tapering off the dose. For a few drugs, this can be extremely difficult, and even require short-term use of other medication. Getting off the tranquilizer Xanax after long-term use can be so difficult it often requires hospitalization. Also, if you're going to quit a drug, you should listen to the doctor's warnings about what risks you will take by stopping. But if the doctor makes quitting sound too scary, maybe it's time to check some other sources (a subject discussed in a later chapter). You're the boss. But follow instructions. Some doctors tell stories about some terrible event that happened when someone stopped taking a drug. For every case where quitting a drug could cause a serious medical problem, there are a hundred where stopping drug treatment will cause little change except to increase your bank balance.

So how do you take charge? Three key resources will provide help: your doctor, your pharmacist, and the drug disclosure label or package insert. The route to being a vigilant, skeptical consumer of drugs is to use all three tools skillfully. Let's examine each briefly:

- Only your doctor has the legal authority to select a drug and write the prescription. As we have seen, doctors are far from infallible. But of all the people whom you can see, doctors have the most extensive training and experience. They are also the only ones who have both information about your medical condition and knowledge of the drugs. But you have the right to know the risks and benefits of the drugs, and the alternatives, including nondrug approaches and forgoing treatment altogether. It is perfectly appropriate and polite to ask your doctor about the risks and benefits of a new medication, or for information about drugs already prescribed. Many doctors have a habit of command; some take little time for questions, and dealing with doctors as a skeptical consumer is something we'll discuss later.

- Pharmacists know a lot about drugs. They have four or more years of specialized training and probably know the medical literature about drugs as well as, or better than, doctors. If you suspect you might be suffering an adverse effect of a drug, or have another factual question about drugs, pharmacists are often the most ready source for a good answer. Most of the time, pharmacists are also approachable and usually welcome questions from customers. Some consumers mistakenly believe their doctors know more than they really do, and underestimate the expertise of their pharmacist.

• The risks and benefits of every prescription drug are described in detail on a document I've been calling the drug disclosure label. It is also called the package insert. You can obtain the disclosure label for any particular drug at your pharmacy. The disclosure labels for many—but not all—modern drugs are collected in a reference volume called the *Physicians' Desk Reference*. The book is almost universally available in libraries and hospitals. Although organized differently, the basic information is also available in a reference book called *Drug Facts and Comparisons*. The problem is that the disclosure labels are written in highly technical language. The sentences are ponderous, long, difficult to read, and include so many forbidding medical terms that at first glance a drug label seems almost impossible to decipher. As noted earlier, some doctors' groups and drug companies have spent fifteen years trying to prevent consumers from getting a simplified, easy-to-read translation. However, the disclosure label is still valuable. I'll explain below how best to use it.

These are the basic tools you'll use to exercise some control over the drugs you're taking. The next step is one everyone should take. You should make a medication register—a summary of the basic facts about every drug you're now taking. (One for every member of your family would be valuable.) Anytime you see a doctor—particularly a specialist or someone new—show the doctor the list. It will help the doctor to select the right drug. Even for those who are not taking any prescription drug now, the same steps apply to your next prescription. The medical register might look like this:

CHEMICAL NAME	BRAND NAME	TABLET SIZE	WHEN TAKEN
conjugated estrogen	Premarin	1.25 mg	Once a day
medroxyprogesterone	Provera	5 mg	1 a day for 10 days each month
ketoprofen	Orudis	75 mg	3 times a day

Also note any special instructions, such as whether to take it with food, or between meals, or at particular times, such as before bedtime.

Most prescription drugs have two names: a complicated chemical, or generic, name; and a short and often catchy brand name. Unfortunately, you'll need to know both names of the drug. The most important name is the chemical name. It identifies the unique chemical molecule in the drug. The chemical name is the same the world over, but brand names vary by country and manufacturer. The chemical name is the only name used in medical journal articles, and it appears more often in news media reports than the brand name. On drug package inserts both names typically appear; however, any mention of other drugs will be by the chemical name. The brand name is a trademarked word that the manufacturer selected to help build name recognition among doctors and consumers. We could just forget about the chemical name except that the brand names are not as reliable and consistent. The same chemical may be marketed under two different brand names. For example the anti-inflammatory drug ketoprofen is sold as Orudis and as Oruvail. Orudis is short-acting ketoprofen that is taken three or four times a day. Oruvail is a sustained-release formulation taken once a day. Generic drugs such as ibuprofen can be sold with just the chemical name, or with brand names such as Advil or Motrin. They're all the same drug. The only term that is consistent, unique, and reliable is the chemical name. The drawback is that the name is typically long, hard to spell, and difficult to pronounce.

Once you've got a list, you should test yourself. For each drug, you ought to be able to say exactly why you're taking the drug, and write it on the paper with the other information about the drugs. It's worth knowing the medical name for your condition. So writing down "hypertension" is better than "high blood pressure," and "angina" is better than "chest pains." If you don't know for certain why you're taking the drug, or have only a vague idea (like "for my heart"), make this a topic for discussion with your doctor. The next step is to look at the patient—that is, yourself.

There is a critical difference between reading this book and talking to a doctor or a pharmacist. A doctor might or might not know all the information in this book. But the doctor should have detailed medical information about your health, and will tailor what he or she says to your particular needs. This book is written for the average reader, in pretty good health, who is taking one or more of the one-to-two hundred most widely prescribed drugs. However, millions of people are not average, and special considerations apply. The next step is to consider whether you are one of these special cases. First, are you one of the 10 percent or more of the population who has experienced unusual reactions to several prescription drugs, maybe to over-the-counter remedies? A little-known biological trait explains why so many of us are a little different. Drugs are typically broken down by the liver, and eliminated from the bloodstream by the kidneys. If you have kidney problems or liver disease, then many drugs are likely to behave quite differently in your system. Unusual drug responses can also occur among heavy drinkers, those who have three or more drinks or glasses of wine, or six or more beers, every day. Also, some of those who are otherwise perfectly normal may nevertheless have unusual responses to drugs. This is because a great many drugs are broken down by special chemicals secreted primarily by the liver, called the P450 system. Most people won't specifically have been told they have abnormal P450 enzymes, but they might have experienced an unusual or extreme adverse reaction to a normal or even very small dose of a drug. The reactions might include becoming extremely nervous, jittery, having heart palpitations or a racing heartbeat. If problems have occurred with one or more drugs, you need to be especially vigilant, and even normal doses may be dangerous.

Second, these chapters are not intended for people with a serious or life-threatening illness—those who have experienced a heart attack, have cancer, epilepsy, juvenile-onset diabetes, multiple sclerosis, or Parkinson's, for example. In such people, the particulars of your medical condition may outweigh the general rules outlined in these chapters. The benefits of drug treatments for serious illness may be much greater (or quite small) and the drug risks often are higher, sometimes very great. (Most drugs for the treatment of cancer are so toxic that their use in reasonably healthy individuals would be unthinkable.) These issues are beyond the scope of these chapters.

The next step in being the boss is to examine the benefits of the drugs you're taking—or of a new prescribed drug. Drugs typically have two kinds of benefits. Some drugs relieve symptoms. They have tangible effects you can feel. Aspirin can make a headache go away, or help with the stiffness in the joints for those with arthritis. If you have a stomach ulcer, then Tagamet or Pepcid may be relieving the pains you are experiencing. Prozac, Zoloft, and Paxil are prescribed to relieve the symptoms of major depression. If you are taking Halcion or Restoril, they should be helping you sleep. For men, Hytrin or Proscar may be relieving the symptoms of prostate problems—or they may be making little or no difference. For these drugs that are supposed to eliminate symptoms, you are the real judge—maybe the only judge—of the benefits. If they don't make you feel better, then maybe you shouldn't be taking them. Often, it's hard to tell whether the drug is working. You injured your left leg in a football game, and after a week on ibuprofen it feels better. Is it healing, or is the drug at work? It may take months before the prostate drug Proscar has any effect on the need to get up at night and urinate, and even then the effect might be very small. For some drugs—for example, the sleep aids Restoril and Halcion—the benefits get smaller and smaller the longer people take them, an effect called tolerance. Not only may these drugs be failing to do their job; they might be making it harder instead of easier to sleep. Other drugs—notably drugs for depression—have mixed effects. Maybe you feel less depressed, but find yourself jittery or having trouble sleeping. Also, for someone suffering through the bleak emotional landscape of depression, feeling jittery may wrongly make them believe, "Gee, this drug is working." A more careful inventory of symptoms and effects may produce evidence that the drug is working or may raise questions about whether the drug is for you.

One of the most common mistakes is for people to take drugs long after they stop needing them. After several months of Tagamet, the ulcer may well have healed and the dramatic benefits may have expired. Tagamet might help prevent a recurrence, but the effects will be much smaller, and you won't feel any different. After a few days or a week on Halcion, the body is making its own adjustments to neutralize the effect of the drug. If you're taking a painkiller, the injury that caused the pain may have healed. So if you're taking a drug that relieves symptoms, there are two key questions. Is the drug clearly helping you feel better? And if you've been taking the drug for weeks or months, do you still need it? Also, most people miss a dose now and then. How do you feel without the drug? (Some drugs persist in the body for days, though, so you won't notice anything if you miss a dose.) Your answer to these questions may be another question. You may not be sure whether you can do without one of these drugs. If so, then this is an issue for a conversation with your doctor—a subject addressed in a later chapter.

For many drugs, the benefits are invisible. If you're taking a drug for mild high blood pressure, it won't produce any effects you can feel, except perhaps for adverse effects. This is also true of people taking drugs to lower their cholesterol, for the mild form of diabetes that doesn't require insulin shots, or estrogen to prevent osteoporosis. Except for adverse effects, the benefits of the drugs are invisible to the patient. You don't feel any different with lower blood sugar, a lower cholesterol level, or lower blood pressure. The purpose of taking these drugs is to prevent injuries, illness, or death. However, as explained earlier, the benefits of drugs given for prevention can be quite small, sometimes benefiting fewer than 1 out of every 100 persons treated for a year. As an individual, you can't tell if the drug has worked. Suppose that after a year of taking a cholesterol-lowering drug you don't have a heart attack. As noted earlier, even without treatment, 90 percent of people with elevated cholesterol won't experience a heart attack in the next five years. Also, you may have a heart attack despite the cholesterol-lowering drug. About 2 out of 3 heart attacks will still occur despite taking cholesterol-lowering drugs, and about 1 out of 2 strokes will still occur despite blood pressure medication. Thus, the major effects of these drugs are invisible to patient and doctor. The theoretical benefits have been determined through scientific experiments with groups of people.

While the benefits of these drugs are invisible, the side effects of many of these drugs may not be. Diuretic drugs for high blood pressure are likely to trigger many extra trips to the bathroom, especially soon after starting the drug. From 10 to 30 percent of people who take medication for high blood pressure will develop side effects severe enough that they will stop taking the drug. However, adjusting the dose or switching the medication can often eliminate the problem. The side effects of cholesterol-lowering drugs run the full spectrum. Drugs such as niacin and Questran have side effects in the majority of the people who take them. (Typically, flushing skin for niacin and digestive problems for Questran.) At the other extreme, only 1 to 3 percent of people taking Pravachol or Zocor experience side effects—usually muscle pains or nausea. When taking drugs for prevention, you should shop for a drug that has no, or minimal, side effects. You should not have to sacrifice the quality of your life to obtain the benefits.

Antibiotics, insulin, and contraceptives are in a class of their own. If given for a proven infection against which the antibiotic is effective, it will be effective about 90 percent of the time. Because these are drugs that cure the medical problem, the effect is on two levels. By solving the underlying medical problem, the medicine also relieves the symptoms. Often, the symptoms go away before the underlying infection is completely eliminated. Consumers frequently make a major mistake with antibiotics and stop taking the drug when the symptoms go away but before the infection has been completely eradicated. This takes us back to lesson number one. You're the boss, but follow instructions. Contraceptives are, of course, better than 99 percent effective in preventing pregnancy. For those with juvenile-onset diabetes, insulin is virtually a 100 percent effective alternative to dying. There are issues you will want to consider in weighing the risks of these drugs, but there are few questions about the benefits.

Returning to the list of drugs, we have now recorded the correct names, the tablet size, and dose of every prescribed drug. We have noted the medical condition being treated and assessed the real benefits of the drug. The next issue is adverse effects. Once again, you are the judge. Some side effects are easy to spot, and start soon after one begins taking a drug. Taking Elavil for depression makes your mouth very dry. Maybe the anti-inflammatory naprosyn upsets your stomach. Or perhaps the diet drug Redux makes you jittery and easily angered. In some people, narcotics for pain trigger hallucinations or severe nausea and vomiting. These are dramatic, rapid-onset adverse effects and the drug is readily identified as the suspect. These side effects usually announce their presence even if you've never been briefed about the specifice adverse effects of the drugs you're taking. In a large majority of cases, these side effects can be eliminated entirely. An adjustment in dose or a switch to another drug often solves the problem—or at least minimizes it. Most of the time, you shouldn't have to tolerate obvious and unpleasant side effects.

The next group of side effects are equally common but often overlooked by patients—and even by doctors. If the adverse effect is subtle, or resembles symptoms you've had before, the drug may not be suspected. For example, I am personally pretty cheerful by nature, and to experience a bout of depression for no identifiable cause would send me on an immediate hunt for a drug or other chemical suspect. Some people have struggled with depression for many years, and they might not blame a new prescription drug. Depression is a common side effect of drugs—not only of the logical suspects such as tranquilizers. It is also caused by blood pressure and cholesterol drugs, by antihistamines, antibiotics, anti-inflammatory drugs, birth control pills, by drugs for irregular heartbeats, epilepsy, and menopause. Scores of other drugs cause similar but milder effects in which people feel listless. The medical term is "asthenia." Major depression is likely to get your attention, but asthenia might be dismissed an "just one of those things." People dismiss such damage to their quality of life as stress or wrongly assume that "I'm just getting older." A depressant effect on the central nervous system is a common side effect frequently overlooked unless it is severe or unusual.

On the other end of the scale, overstimulation or anxiety is another easily overlooked adverse effect. Hundreds of drugs can cause this problem. Overstimulation occurs with drugs one might not normally suspect. For example, it is a very common effect of Imitrex, the drug for migraine headache; it occurs with Accutane for acne, and the broad spectrum antibiotics such as Floxin, Cipro, and Noroxin. Even doctors may not be aware that drugs intended to calm anxiety make it worse in some patients, and drugs for depression sometimes make the depression worse. Persistent itching, skin rash, or hives are so common and familiar that people may not suspect a drug—yet these are among the most common adverse effects of drugs. The heart is another target organ for drug adverse effects. Palpitations or a rapid heartbeat are a very common adverse effect of numerous drugs.

Another group of side effects may begin with mild symptoms but signal a major medical problem that requires immediate attention. One warning sign is persistent nausea that might begin weeks or months after starting a drug. This reaction can be a symptom of liver damage and needs immediate medical attention. One strategy for dealing with the more subtle symptoms will be outlined later. A cut that doesn't heal, or a sore throat that won't go away, or repeated infections are other mild symptoms of an extremely serious adverse drug reaction. These problems may be the only symptoms of a drug that is destroying your white blood cells. If you find you bruise too easily, or bleeding does not stop, these are warning signs for other blood cell disorders. You should make an immediate trip to your doctor for a blood test. This is not intended to be a list of all the symptoms that might signal the adverse effects of drugs. Rather, these common mild symptoms can be easily overlooked. If you encounter a specific medical problem—or just find yourself without your normal health and energy—consider drugs as a possible suspect.

The third and last kind of side effect is detected only through the vigilance of your doctor, because by the time there are definite symptoms, the medical situation is very serious. Many widely used drugs fall into this category and require medical monitoring to detect the adverse effects. For example, one family of cholesterol-lowering drugs—including Mevacor, Zocor, and Pravachol—may damage the liver. The evidence of the liver damage can be observed by laboratory tests on a blood sample. For patients on these medications, the doctor is supposed to check for liver damage six and twelve weeks after first starting this drug and twice a year thereafter. The anticlotting agent Coumadin is another drug requiring constant medical vigilance. While the drug is capable of preventing painful blood clots from forming in the legs and helps prevents strokes, a small overdose is dangerous, causing bleeding. The doctor needs to order laboratory tests of your bleeding time and blood-clotting function to make sure the dose is right. The tests should be repeated anytime you take a new drug or make a major change in your diet. Here is another reason for having a master list of the medications you're taking. By the time your toes turn purple (a clear symptom of a Coumadin overdose), it is possible that gangrene may have already occurred. Lanoxin—the most frequently prescribed heart drug—is a third example of a drug requiring physician vigilance to prevent adverse effect. Preventing a dangerous overdose may require blood tests to measure the concentration of the drug, a check of kidney function, and the effect of other commonly prescribed drugs. It's important to know whether you're taking a drug that requires special medical vigilance. Unfortunately, about the only way to find out that information is to check a drug reference, or the product's disclosure label. A later chapter will explain how to get what you need to know out of the forbidding drug label information.

CHAPTER THIRTEEN

Getting the Facts

HERE IS AN IMPORTANT warning about adverse effects of Vasotec, the best-selling blood pressure drug in the United States in 1995. It comes from the package insert, or product disclosure label:

WARNINGS:

ANAPHYLACTOID AND POSSIBLY RELATED REACTIONS Presumably because angiotensin-converting enzyme inhibitors affect the metabolism of eicosanoids and polypeptides, including endogenous bradykinin, patients receiving ACE inhibitors (including VASOTEC) may be subject to a variety of adverse reactions, some of them serious.

Fortunately, this is one of the worst examples of the unreadable language in which drug disclosure labels are written. In plain English, it says that Vasotec (like penicillin) can trigger allergic reactions, and that sometimes these allergic reactions are serious. However, as we begin to explore the valuable information buried in drug disclosure labels, the best approach is not to be intimidated. As far as I can tell, the only reason for writing these documents in such unreadable language is to draw as little attention as possible to drug dangers while taking credit for having forthrightly disclosed their risks. (Even most doctors couldn't tell you much about "the metabolism of eicosanoids.") Thanks to the concerted effort of doctors' groups and drug companies described earlier, a simple and accurate English-language translation of the drug disclosure label is not readily available. So it will take some time, patience, a medical dictionary, and this chapter. To be your own boss, it is essential to know something about the drugs you're taking. Anyone who completes this short course in reading a drug label is likely to discover something surprising and useful about practically any drug that is checked. This chapter also provides a checklist of questions to ask about every prescription drug. The disclosure label is where the answers are located.

A word of encouragement. This task may seem impossibly complex at first. But break the job down into smaller, simple steps, and you'll be amazed at your progress.

A drug disclosure label is a reference document; it is not like a short story or book that needs to be read from the beginning. Like a dictionary, a label is an excellent source of answers to specific questions. The label is organized so readers can find the same information in the same place on every label. A dictionary organizes the material in alphabetical order; a drug label has a different plan, but equally predictable. Most of the answers can be found in the disclosure label. We'll focus most on the information you're not likely to get from the regular sources. (For example, most people know how much of the drug to take, and how many times a day to take it.) In exploring the drug label, let's keep a reasonable goal clearly in view. This book chapter, or any book chapter, can't provide enough background to permit you to assess authoritatively the risks and benefits of a particular drug. However, in almost every case the reader should find (and this is worth the trouble) nuggets of gold—important questions worth pursuing with the doctor or pharmacist. Even if you find nothing to worry about, it's still reassuring to know you've made all the prudent checks.

Before answering specific questions—or mining the gold in the disclosure labels—let's begin with an assault on the major obstacle, the difficult medical language. If you or a family member take drugs routinely or have medical problems, it is worth investing in a medical dictionary. As someone who ten years ago started to read medical studies without formal training, I continue to be amazed at the simple statements that are cloaked in complex medical jargon. If your hair falls out, it is called alopecia; an inflamed liver becomes "hepatitis," and an allergy is described as "anaphylactoid and possibly related reactions." Translated back into simple English, what first looked impossibly complicated turns out to be striaghtforward and readily understandable. The doctors and researchers insist on using their own very specific language and spend the better part of two years in medical school mastering it. The layman needs to learn only a few medical terms. It's the difference between knowing enough French to find the public bathroom in Paris and writing a dissertation about the French Revolution. For the medical tourist, the best solution is to wait until you encounter a word you need to know and then look it up.

A handful of medical terms appear so often and describe such basic ideas that it is worth knowing them from the start. These terms describe bedrock concepts of drugs and the medical conditions they address, and are worth knowing in their own right. The first two deal with a key concept of drug safety.

Acute. Means sudden onset, often an emergency. An acute episode of asthma means a sudden difficulty breathing. The next term helps define it by contrast.

Chronic. Means long-term or persistent; something that doesn't go away.

Acute and chronic effects are basic to the nature of both diseases and the drugs intended to combat them. Asthma can be a *chronic* condition, meaning that is is a medical problem that can last for years. Those suffering from asthma also have acute episodes. One drug (such as Serevent) is prescribed for the chronic condition. An entirely different drug (for example, Proventil) is used for an acute episode. Both are given through an inhaler. A cholesterol-lowering drug might be prescribed to deal with the chronic problem of slowly developing heart disease. For an acute episode of chest pains, you pop a nitroglycerin pill under your tongue. Some drugs are designed to cope with acute episodes. (Nitroglycerin will stop chest pains, aspirin will reduce the pain of an inflamed tendon.) Other drugs are intended for treating chronic disease. It can be dangerous—even lethal—to attempt to cope with an acute episode by taking an extra dose of a drug designed for slow, long-term chronic effect. For example, taking extra doses from a Serevent inhaler can kill you. Not only does everyone need to know what these words mean; you should know whether the drugs you take can be used for acute episodes.

Hypersensitivity, anaphylaxis, anaphylactoid. These words describe allergic reactions. Drugs are designed to elude the immune system defense, which is continually on guard to identify and attack foreign substances that get into the body—especially viruses and microbes. With some drugs, and in some people, the immune system learns to recognize the peculiar-shaped molecules of a prescription drug and mounts an attack. Typically, an allergic reaction has two phases. Little or nothing happens the first time a person is exposed. However, after about three days the immune system has identified the drug as an invader and is preparing a massive response if it ever encounters that molecule again. This is the situation in which the really dangerous allergic reactions occur. This also means, unfortunately, that you can't be sure you have no drug allergies from a single administration of a drug. After exposure, the allergic reaction is sometimes a mild response—for example, a skin rash, redness, or swelling. Occasionally, a massive immune response gets out of control—a condition called anaphylaxis or anaphylactic shock. Swelling can be so severe and pervasive it can block the airways and be fatal. Penicillin is the best-known example of a drug likely to trigger an allergic reaction. But other drugs (for example, Vasotec, Prinivil, Captopril and other blood pressure drugs called ACE inhibitors) often cause allergic effects. Literally thousands of drug labels warn doctors not to give this drug to people known to be "hypersensitive" to it. This is just a commonsense warning that anyone would follow: Don't take anything you're allergic to.

Rare, infrequent. These words appear routinely on drug disclosure labels. They almost always describe adverse effects. The problem is that the term "rare" is not used consistently. In labels, "rare" is supposed to mean "observed in fewer than 1 in 1,000 cases." However, in some cases "rare" has been used to describe a common adverse effect of a drug, affecting 1 or 2 percent of those who take it. Compounding this sloppy use of language is another major problem described earlier. Less than 1 percent of adverse reactions are reported either to the manufacturer or the FDA. The adverse effect could therefore be much more common than stated. Even if the manufacturer honestly believes the adverse effect is rare based on the handful of reports it has received, many more people could have been affected. Except to compare two different drugs, you may not care about how frequent an adverse effect may be. If you don't have the problem, then it may not be important to you how many other people suffer. If you do have this symptom, the rarity of the event is of little interest. Even if only 1 in 10,000 people is affected, the problem is of great importance if the victim is you. It might make the drug manufacturer feel better to know the problem its product causes is "rare." But it won't make you feel better until you eliminate that side effect with a change in dosage, a change in drug, or a halt in therapy.

Also, just because an adverse effect is reported to be infrequent doesn't mean you should dismiss the drug as a suspect. (Unfortunately, it might make it harder to convince a doctor who hasn't seen a case before.) So when examining the listed adverse effects, the frequency is not very important. You want the longest possible list to see whether the drug is a logical suspect for why you're not feeling your usual self. The classic test of whether a drug is responsible for an adverse effect is to stop the drug and see if the adverse effect disappears. Then drug treatment is resumed; if the side effect reappears, this is a strong indication the drug is responsible. This test—called a rechallenge—requires a doctor's assistance.

Now it's time to examine the drug disclosure label directly. Labels are divided into ten sections. (A few have an extra section or two, or are missing one.) Some sections can be routinely ignored; others deserve careful study. The first priority is to look for warnings. Check the package insert for warnings even if you decide not to study it further. Generally, warnings report problems that are serious enough that they might influence the decision whether or not to take a drug. Almost every drug has a warning section. (The ulcer drug Zantac is apparently so benign that it doesn't have any warnings.) Warnings on a drug label are something like the headlines on the front page of a newspaper; the most important stories are highlighted through bigger type and more prominent placement.

PAY ATTENTION! The most draconian drug warnings are placed in boldface capital letters and enclosed in a box at the very top of the disclosure label, where they will be easily seen. Here is an example, from Premarin:[1]

---

1. ESTROGENS HAVE BEEN REPORTED TO INCREASE THE RISK OF ENDOMETRIAL CARCINOMA. Three independent, case-controlled studies have reported an increased risk of endometrial cancer in post-menopausal women exposed to exogenous estrogens for more than one year.
2. ESTROGENS SHOULD NOT BE USED DURING PREGNANCY. The use of female sex hormones, both estrogens and progestogens, during pregnancy may seriously damage the offspring.

The warning on the actual Premarin label is a little more detailed. But the message here is readable and clear. Never take sex hormones during pregnancy, and beware of the cancer risk with long-term use. Sometimes the box is not at the top of the drug label, but it will still stand out. If you see any bold black type enclosed in a box, read that first. Occasionally, the black type at the beginning of the disclosure label may say **Caution** instead of **Warning**. Still, pay careful attention.

WARNINGS. Drug labels also have a regular warning section with this heading, usually in the middle of the text. It is organized just like the stories in a local newspaper. The most important fact or facts come first, with less important material below. **IF IT IS REALLY IMPORTANT, IT IS IN BOLD-FACE CAPITALS.** Such warnings usually apply to the most horrifying drug risks—dangers such as death, cancer, cardiac arrest, destruction of the bone marrow, or birth defects. One of the mildest examples is the warning for the antibiotic tetracycline. It can permanently discolor children's teeth. If this antibiotic was prescribed for your eight-year-old child, you should go back to the doctor immediately. **Important warnings are in boldface.** They usually describe life-threatening conditions, but perhaps they can be managed with prompt medical attention. A serious allergic reaction is an example. Other less severe warnings are in regular type. The first step in reading a drug label is to check the warnings. A large number of drugs (about 2,300), have routine warnings that you should not take this drug if you are allergic to it. But for those drugs with serious risks, the hazard is clearly identified in a more prominent warning.

INDICATIONS AND USAGE. Vital safety information is contained in this section of every drug label. Many consumers would be reluctant to take a drug that is not FDA-approved. (At least they should be. At the very least, the skeptical consumer ought to do some extra checking.) However, FDA approval has a very important limitation. Approval really means that the FDA has certified that a drug is effective for a specific medical purpose. That specific medical purpose is called the "indication." It is described in this section of the drug label. If the drug is prescribed or used for any other purpose—an unfortunately frequent event—you are outside the FDA umbrella of protection. The FDA-approved indication is a key safety concept everyone should know. The FDA stamp of approval applies only to the specific medical use described on the drug disclosure label. Just as everyone should be familiar with the important warnings, it is essential to know whether the drug has been subject to the full rigor of FDA-required scientific testing for your specific medical problem.

The question, therefore, is whether your own medical condition is described as an approved indication for the drug. For example, Vasotec is indicated for "the treatment of hypertension." The Prozac label says the drug "is indicated for the treatment of depression." The indication for ibuprofen shows it was tested and found effective "for the temporary relief of minor aches and pains associated with the common cold, headache, toothache, muscular aches, backache, for the minor pain of arthritis, for the pain of menstrual cramps, and for reduction of fever." If the indication describes your medical condition, this is just the reassurance you want. But suppose you were prescribed Lopid (or gemfibrozil), a best-selling drug for high cholesterol. A reading of the indication would raise warning flags immediately. In the indications section is this message (boldface capitals in the original):

BECAUSE OF POTENTIAL TOXICITY SUCH AS MALIGNANCY, GALLBLADDER DISEASE, ABDOMINAL PAIN LEADING TO APPENDECTOMY AND OTHER ABDOMINAL SURGERIES, AN INCREASED INCIDENCE IN NONCORONARY MORTALITY, AND THE 44% RELATIVE INCREASE DURING THE TRIAL PERIOD IN AGE-ADJUSTED ALL-CAUSE MORTALITY SEEN WITH THE CHEMICALLY AND PHARMACOLOGICALLY RELATED DRUG CLOFIBRATE, THE POTENTIAL BENEFIT OF GEMFIBROZIL IN TREATING TYPE IIA PATIENTS WITH ELEVATIONS OF LDL-CHOLESTEROL ONLY IS NOT LIKELY TO OUTWEIGH THE RISKS.

This sentence says the FDA has concluded the benefit of Lopid "is not likely to outweigh the risks" for patients who have the typical form of high cholesterol, elevated levels of LDL (or bad) cholesterol. Lopid is indicated only for a rare lipid abnormality. In fact, the FDA found that Parke-Davis, the manufacturer of Lopid, had violated the regulations by advertising this drug for more general-purpose cholesterol lowering. The FDA required corrective advertising in medical journals, but not before hundreds of thousands of patients ended up taking this drug for an indication that the FDA declares is inappropriate. It is not unusual to survey the indications section and find other examples where use "is not recommended" or "should be avoided." This is an issue you will want to pursue. The next chapter will describe how to do so.

Already we have seen one of the best-kept secrets of the indications section. It defines the specific medical conditions for which the drug received the FDA stamp of approval, which is awarded only after rigorous clinical testing. Any other uses of the drug are, in some fashion, experimental and have higher risk. The indications section of some drug labels contains language intended to send up another kind of warning flag for those who know how to read it. As noted many times in this book, FDA approval does not mean that a drug is safe and can be used freely without concern. FDA approval means that a drug has been tested thoroughly enough to be proven effective for certain medical uses. But we have already seen that some approved drugs are extremely toxic, and even the most common drugs, such as aspirin and ibuprofen, cause severe injuries in some. While the public thinks of drug approval as a yes-or-no decision, the FDA actually crafts the indications section as carefully as a writer labors over the opening paragraph of a new book. As safety concerns about a drug mount, one FDA response is ever more prominent label warnings—like the black box for Premarin. The other strategy is to narrow the indication, or approved use, of the drug. This doesn't stop doctors form prescribing the drug as they please. However, checking the indications section tells the consumer whether FDA safety experts had reservations about this drug but still approved it. The FDA safety concern that is most easily spotted by a reader without a medical background is called a "second-line indication." It means the FDA advises using this drug only if other drugs have already failed. It says that for most patients a safer alternative is available. Here is an example of the section for a once extremely popular antibiotic, chloramphenicol, or Chloromycetin:

INDICATIONS AND USAGE:
In accord with the concepts in the warning box and this indications section, Chloramphenicol must be used only in those serious infections for which less potentially dangerous drugs are ineffective or contraindicated.

Clearly, the FDA is saying, "Avoid this drug if possible."

Here is another example of a second-line indication, for an AIDS drug that is similar to AZT:

INDICATIONS AND USAGE:
Zerit™ (Stavudine) capsules is indicated for treatment of adults with advanced HIV infection who are intolerant of approved therapies with proven clinical benefit or who have experienced significant clinical or immunologic deterioration while receiving these therapies or for whom such therapies are contraindicated.

In plain English, this label says don't use Zerit unless the patient is already in serious trouble and everything else has failed. Zerit was a drug the AIDS community was clamoring for. In testing Zerit, the same dose that proved barely effective in the major clinical study was rejected as too toxic in a separate safety study.[2] In what was not one of its better days, the FDA approved Zerit with the recommendation that patients should avoid it if at all possible.

The larger point is that any language in the indications section saying that other drugs should be tried first is a major warning flag. If other alternatives have not been tried before a second-line drug was prescribed, this is an issue to take up with your doctor. (Using second-line drugs without trying first-line drugs is another example of inappropriate prescribing.)

Sometimes you will find your medical problem described plainly in the indications section. This is comforting evidence you are under the full umbrella of protection provided by FDA approval. Occasionally, there will be a direct warning, such as for Lopid, to avoid this drug except for certain medical conditions. Frequently, however, you will find nothing in the indications section that even remotely applies to your medical condition. Welcome to the untidy world of "off-label" drug use. A drug company can advertise and promote a drug only for its FDA-approved indication, the medical purpose for which it was tested. Physicians, however, have latitude to prescribe drugs as they see fit, subject only to the check of outright malpractice. No matter how much or how little testing might have been done, physicians may experiment on their patients with medical uses for which the drug was not approved by the FDA. In some cases, these off-label uses are widely accepted in the medical community and based on sound clinical research. The only thing missing is the formal step of FDA approval and inclusion on the drug label. In other cases, these off-label uses became widely accepted in medicine but were never properly tested by anyone. This is what happened when doctors used Tambocor, Enkaid, and other drugs to treat very mild irregular heartbeats. The drugs were not FDA-approved for this purpose, and not only were the drugs ineffective, but they caused cardiac arrest. The widespread off-label use is a great weakness in the system. Unfortunately, if you can't find your own medical problem listed among the approved indications, you'll have to inquire elsewhere to find out why you've been prescribed a drug for off-label use.

Off-label use is the rule rather than the exception in several situations. At least half, and possibly a majority, of cancer patients are prescribed at least one drug for an unapproved, off-label use. Because anticancer drugs don't work very well, experimentation is common with cancer patients. In other cases, oncologists try drugs that have been proven effective against one cancer in the hope they will work against another.

Children are another special case. Drugs are seldom tested separately in children, even though drugs sometimes have different effects in children than in adults.* Drugs for depression, for example, have failed repeatedly to provide teenagers and other young people the benefits seen in adults.[3] Some doctors still prescribe them even though they are not indicated for this age group and probably don't work. In other cases, we assume they are safe in children; physicians adjust the dose for the smaller body weight, and everyone hopes for the best. It is all we can get out of a safety system that does not require testing in children. But in both cases, the consumer should not be surprised to discover off-label use.

The consumer should also be wary of off-label use of drugs for cholesterol lowering, blood pressure, estrogen or other hormones. More than a hundred drugs are approved for hy-

---

*As this book goes to press, the FDA has proposed to require that some drugs be tested in children. If finalized, this initiative would improve this situation in a few years.

pertension and several dozen for high cholesterol. It is hard to imagine the need for risking a drug with less than the full umbrella of FDA approval. Another situation to check carefully is when you have a mild condition and discover a label indication that says this drug is only for serious cases. The classic example is drugs for severe mental illness such as schizophrenia. As noted before, these drugs carry major risks of brain damage and severe injury; individuals with anxiety or depression ought to inquire carefully before taking them. An unwritten and somewhat frightening rule applies to drugs for the most serious illnesses. The medical community has proved willing to accept very high levels of toxicity for the most serious illnesses and low levels of effectiveness. This is notably true of drugs for cancer and mental illness. This occurs, I believe, because in such grave situations doctors feel compelled to try something. "First Do No Harm"—the golden rule of medicine—is too often replaced by the modern medical commandment, "At Least Try Something." If you don't have a serious illness, and discover you are prescribed a drug normally reserved for such situations, check with great care the need for this drug and whether there are safer substitutes. (For example, I was amazed to discover that Haldol, a powerful and dangerous antipsychotic drug with grave risks, is routinely prescribed as a sedative and sleep aid.)[4]

CONTRAINDICATIONS. This section describes the people who should not take this drug. Contraindications are so serious that if you believe this section of the label applies to you, don't take the drug again until you have talked to your doctor or pharmacist. The purpose of this section of the drug label is straightforward and unambiguous: For these people the dangers of the drug outweigh its possible benefits. They shouldn't take this drug. A classic contraindication is for Trimox, Wymox, Amoxil, Augmentin, or other brands of the best-selling antibiotic amoxicillin. Anyone with a history of any penicillin allergy shouldn't take even one pill without checking further. Another example is the beta-blocker Inderal for people with asthma. This otherwise valuable heart drug can make asthma much worse. Because birth control pills can cause blood clots and stroke, they shouldn't be used by people with a history of such problems. Checking the contraindications is simple and easy. The section is short—a few sentences—and explicit. If you find an entry that might apply to you, check with a pharmacist or doctor before taking any more of this drug.

The warnings, the indications, and the contraindications summarize the headline news on drug disclosure labels, with the really important facts displayed in boldface or boldface capitals. However, the other sections of the label may provide useful detail, and for some people, vital information. The next section of the drug label to check is "Precautions." When the system is working right, the essential precautions have been elevated to a warning or prominently displayed elsewhere. Nevertheless, the precautions section is useful because you can always find certain information here.

If you are a woman who is pregnant, or might get pregnant, the precautions section contains a summary of the drug's risk. Look in the precautions section of the drug label for the heading "Pregnancy" or "Pregnancy/Teratongenic Effects." For once, it has been made easy, because immediately after that heading comes the pregnancy category with this simple letter rating system.

Pregnancy Category[5]

A = Evidence of safety from human testing

B = No evidence of harm in animal testing

C = Harm in animal testing or untested

D = Evidence of harm in humans
X = Pregnant women strongly advised to avoid

Unfortunately, the disclosure label does not explain what the letter ratings mean. Even reference volumes such as the *Physicians' Desk Reference* don't explain them. But the meanings are as described above. The official regulation that defines these letter ratings says that in Category C the drugs may be used "Only if benefits outweigh the risk." In Category D, the drugs should be used "only if life threatening situations or for a serious disease."[6] Even if you're a man, or not pregnant, it might be worth checking the pregnancy category of the drug. It's a very crude indication of overall toxicity in the sense that the most benign drugs are also likely to be Class A or B. In a system designed to inform consumers instead of keeping them in the dark, other drug risks would be reported in simple-to-understand ratings. An 'A" could mean a drug with very low toxicity. A "D" could mean "Watch out! This is a dangerous drug." Just after the pregnancy category in the precautions section is a highly technical discussion of the research results in animal testing that led to assigning the rating.

Drug interactions are the next item to check in the precautions section. You'll need to know the chemical names—not the brand names—of the other drugs you're taking. The last chapter described how to make a list, which will now prove handy. Only a few drug interactions set off all the urgent alarm bells. (Like taking Hismanal and Nizoral, the antifungal agent.) A more typical drug interaction report will say that the drug "might" make another drug more potent, or reduce its effectiveness. If you are taking two potentially interacting drugs, this is another item to draw to the attention of your doctor and to note on your register of drugs. If you've experienced an adverse effect, an interaction might be causing an overdose. A dose adjustment might eliminate the problem.

The precautions section also contains the information about the cancer risks of drugs. Unlike the easy-to-read pregnancy risk categories, the cancer risk findings are usually difficult to read. The cancer testing results are summarized under a standard heading entitled "Carcinogenesis, Mutagenesis, and Impairment of Fertility." For a very few drugs, a clear, English-language warning will appear. For example, the disclosure label for Climara, which is estrogen for menopausal women dispensed through a skin patch, is in plain English: "Long-term continuous administration of natural and synthetic estrogens in certain animal species increases the frequency of carcinomas of the breasts, uterus, cervix, vagina, testis, and liver." (Like other estrogen drugs, it also has the boxed warning quoted above.) Such clear and readable statements about cancer risk are rare. More usual is this statement about the cancer risks of Pravachol (or pravastatin) the best-selling cholesterol drug:

> In a 2-year study in rats fed pravastatin at doses of 10, 30, or 100 mg/kg body weight, there was an increased incidence of hepatocellular carcinomas in males at the highest dose ($p<0.01$). Although rats were given up to 125 times the human dose (HD) on a mg/kg body weight basis, serum drug levels were only 6 to 10 times higher than those measured in humans given 40 mg pravastatin as measured by AUC.

In plain English, the manufacturer says Pravachol caused liver cancer in rats at doses that were six to ten times higher than recommended for humans. (But the rats were only given Pravachol for two years while humans might take it for ten years.) If you kept reading, the label would say a chemically similar drug caused cancer in a second animal species, mice. So how does an average, well-informed consumer interpret these scientific data? The truth is that no one knows exactly what this means. The earlier chapter about cancer risks noted two key facts: For millions of people, prescription drugs are their greatest exposure to chemicals with the potential to cause cancer. About half of all approved drugs carry some cancer risk. Pravachol falls in that group of potentially carcinogenic drugs. On the other hand, in absolute terms, the risks are relatively small. One of the best-established human carcinogens yet identified—estrogen—caused endometrial cancer in 5 out of every 1,000 women exposed for more than five years. (Among asbestos workers and heavy smokers, lung cancer occurred in 4 out of every 1,000 people each year.) In my own view, the capacity to cause cancer weighs the balance against a drug, but unless I had medical reason to be very concerned about cancer risk, I personally would not reject a drug only because of its cancer risk in animal studies. But it could be the third strike to call the drug out, or weigh in the balance, especially for drugs you expect to take for many years.

Given that even the experts don't know the meaning of these studies reported on the drug label, the skeptical consumer can take a simple approach. For about half the drugs, the carcinogenesis section will say no evidence was found. For example, the label for the antiulcer drug Zantac says: "There was no indication of tumorigenic or carcinogenic effects in life-span studies in mice and rats at dosages up to 2,000 mg per day." When a drug gets a clean bill of health on cancer risks, it is usually expressed in readable fashion. Almost any observed abnormalities, even reports of benign growths are warning flags of some cancer risk. (That's because every chemical agent known to produce benign growths also produces some outright cancers.) The cancer risk section will also report whether the drug caused cell mutations—another strong indication of cancer risk because the genetic material of the cells is damaged. Fortunately, not too many drugs fail this test.

Almost all the drug labels have cancer risk sections. A notable exception are the best-selling penicillin drugs, Trimox, Amoxil, and other forms of amoxicillin. These drugs were approved before the FDA requirements for the standard battery of cancer tests that now apply to every drug.

The precautions section contains other useful information. As noted earlier, some drugs require laboratory tests or other special vigilance by your doctor. Mevacor, Zocor, and Pravachol require regular blood tests to check for liver damage. Other drugs need lab checks for signs of damage to the bone marrow, or to gauge drug effects on blood clotting. In some cases, the same oral dose may produce quite different concentrations in the bloodstream in different individuals. This may require monitoring blood concentrations to adjust the dose. The precautions section will describe any necessary testing. Don't worry if the description of the test is hard to understand. You don't have to do the test yourself. You should note, however, whether some form of ongoing testing is required. I couldn't find any studies on this subject, but doctors tell me that failure to do the follow-up testing is as common a failing as outright prescribing error.

ADVERSE REACTIONS. This section is the next stop. The lengthy and forbidding list of potential problems is about as interesting to read as a telephone book and should be used the same way—to look up the information you want. In the adverse reaction section, the readability of label information reaches a new low. Simple and common problems, such as being without normal energy and vigor, are concealed behind mysterious medical language—in this case the term "asthenia." Serious and alarming effects, such as brain damage to areas controlling the voluntary muscles, have cryptic medical names, in this case, "tardive dyskinesia." On different drug labels, the same basic problem may be described with different words. For example, as noted earlier, many, many drugs can overstimulate the central nervous system. Think about the worst case of overstimulation you can remember—maybe the day you were already excited and then drank much too much coffee. However, depending on the drug, this might be described as agitation, anxiety, CNS (central nervous system) stimulation, excitability, feeling shaky, insomnia, jitteriness, hyperactivity, talkativeness, or trembling. There is no uniform vocabulary for describing adverse effects.[7]

A retired FDA medical officer named John Nestor told me about a deliberate industry trick he would sometimes notice while reviewing drug-testing results. Suppose a company became concerned that their drug had produced 100 cases of overstimulation of the nervous system in clinical trials and feared this would draw too many questions from the FDA. Some companies would try to minimize the drug's problems by dividing up the cases into smaller categories. For example, the 100 cases might be divided into 20 cases of jitteriness, 10 cases of excitability, and so forth. My advice is not to try to make sense out of the long lists in the adverse reactions section. If you have a problem you think a drug might cause, see if you can find it listed. Your search can be substantially narrowed because the adverse effects are listed by body system. A problem related to an upset stomach will be listed under "Digestive System," itching or a skin rash under "Skin and Appendages."

Sometimes the adverse reaction section will summarize the adverse reactions detected in the clinical testing required for FDA approval. Here is part of the table for Paxil:

BODY SYSTEM	PREFERRED TERM	PAXIL (N=421)	PLACEBO (N= 421)
Body as a whole	Headache	18%	17%
	Asthenia	15%	6%
Urogenital system	Ejaculatory disturbances	13%	0%

A table such as this is more informative, but take care not to overestimate the adverse effects caused by the drug. The first entry shows that 18 percent of the 421 Paxil patients reported a headache. Should you blame those headaches on Paxil? There's no evidence in here that Paxil causes headaches. If you look at the placebo patients—who thought they were taking Paxil but actually got an inactive pill—about the same number (17 percent) had headaches. Thus, check the results among patients on a placebo before blaming the drug. Now let's look at the third adverse effect, "ejaculatory disturbances." In this case 13 percent of those on Paxil reported this problem, but 0 percent of those on placebos. No doubt here that Paxil can affect sexual functioning in men. For the second side effect, asthenia, or depleted vitality, the results were different again. Some of the placebo patients (6 percent) didn't feel their usual selves (we all have bad days) but more than twice as many treated patients had the problem. In this case, suspect a real effect. A general rule is that the day-to-day discomforts that we all feel—upset stomachs, headaches, depleted vitality, dizziness—are often found as frequently among placebo patients. The drug is to blame only if there is a substantial excess. Other adverse effects are really quite rare and will seldom occur unless the drug (or something substantial) is causing it. This includes items such as the sexual problems reported by the men taking Paxil, sleeplessness for several days, or perversion of the sense of taste.

If you're feeling fine now—or if you have a newly prescribed drug—a more cursory look at the adverse effects ought to suffice. Does the drug have a lengthy list of adverse effects, or are only a few listed? Check whether the drug is likely to affect your behavior: Can it make you feel anxious or groggy, impair judgment or thinking? If one day soon you're not feeling or acting like your usual self, it's nice to be able to rule out the prescription drug in the search for a cause. Some people may have an adverse affect that would be of special concern. If you're recovering from infectious hepatitis, it might be worth checking for possible effects on the liver; if you have heart problems, check cardiovascular effects. If you don't have any special medical problems, I'm not sure how much you gain by studying the fine details of what might happen to you, any more than it helps to be morbidly concerned about being struck by lightning, run over by a car, or getting cancer. The main role of the adverse reaction list is to check out suspects if a problem occurs.

DOSAGE AND ADMINISTRATION. Your last job is to check and think about the dose. For many drugs, the right dose is the key to getting the benefits without suffering adverse effects. It is also time to return to the message of the last chapter and remember: You are the boss, but follow instructions. You can't get a prescription without a doctor. You can't change to another drug without a doctor. But millions of people do stop taking drugs or increase the dose in hopes of increasing the effect. (Some people, but many fewer, reduce the dose.) Sometimes that's a reasonable course of action. With other drugs, a unilateral change in dose is extremely risky. While the dose happens to fall under the patient's control, the dose can be just as critical an element of success or failure as getting the right drug, or a correct diagnosis. In some cases, the instructions that come with the prescription say that you can and should alter the dose (within specified limits) to get the best effect. An asthma inhaler such as Ventolin is designed to be used that way. But someone taking theophylline tablets for asthma could be taking grave risks by increasing the dose.

With certain drugs, it's almost as if a black line is painted on the floor. You are pretty safe until you cross it, then watch out! The classic example is Tylenol, or acetaminophen. It is used in hospitals and as the first choice drug for arthritis because it doesn't have the same risk of causing ulcers and intestinal bleeding as aspirin, ibuprofen, and similar anti-inflammatory drugs. In short, it seems safer. But at about two and a half times the recommended dose of Extra-Strength Tylenol, the drug can become extremely toxic to the liver—even destroy it with lethal effect. In those whose liver may be damaged by years of heavy alcohol consumption, toxic effects can occur at an even lower dose. On the other hand, someone who takes two and a half times the typical dose of aspirin will be taking only a little more than the amount used by people with severe arthritis. In many cases, acetaminophen is a safer bet than as-pirin, but don't fool around with the dose. If it doesn't do the job, maybe it is time for another painkiller. In most cases, you will need a doctor's help to adjust the dose.

Tolerance is the next potential dose issue. Maybe it takes an extra Xanax to produce the exact same calming effect. You take an extra Vicodin to live with the pain in your knee. Some drugs reliably produce the same effect, year in and year out. In others, the body regards the chemical control changes made by the drug as undesirable and slowly makes adjustments to neutralize their effect. As described in the earlier section about addiction, tolerance also means that adverse effects can occur when the dose is reduced. For decades, barbiturates such as Nembutal and phenobarbital were a tolerance death trap that claimed thousands of lives. People took ever increasing amounts to maintain the same effect in calming anxiety or promoting sleep. Also, alcohol enhanced the depressant effect greatly. Thousands of people slowly increased the dose until they took enough to kill themselves. A higher dose and extra drinks with dinner was all it took. In most drugs in which tolerance is a potential problem, a notice will appear in the warnings section. But any time you sense you need a higher dose to achieve the same effect, that should set off warning bells.

The last step is easy. With these precautions in mind, check whether the amount prescribed falls in the recommended dosage range. Typically the recommended doses are listed as the total amount per day in milligrams. Here is the section for Prozac (or fluoxetine):

Depression: Initial Treatment—In controlled trials used to support the efficacy of fluoxetine, patients were administered morning doses ranging from 20 mg to 80 mg/day. Studies comparing fluoxetine 20, 40 and 60 mg/day to placebo indicate that 20 mg/day is sufficient to obtain a satisfactory antidepressant response in most cases.

To figure how much you're taking, check the medicine bottle to find out the tablet size. This information is essential to making the right calculation. (The last section, "How Supplied," also tells the tablet sizes in which the drug is available.) Prozac is available in both 10 mg and 20 mg tablets. So instructions to take two tablets in the morning could be 20 mg a day if you received the 10 mg tablets, or 40 mg a day if you were prescribed the larger tablets.

If you discover that you might be taking a dose outside the therapeutic range, take the medicine bottle to the pharmacist and ask him or her to help you check. If because of tolerance you have marched up to or exceeded the maximum dose, it's time to see your doctor. Generally, you want the lowest effective dose. The other reason to check the dose is a possible mistake, a prescribing or dispensing error. In hospitals (where this is studied most carefully) a prescribing error occurs with chilling regularity. A 1997 study of an Albany, New York, hospital found a 3 to 4 percent chance that a hospitalized patient would fall victim to an error in writing the prescription.[8] Almost half the mistakes made were overdoses. That is good enough reason to check for yourself. In hospitals, one of the most common errors is a misplaced decimal point that results in getting a dose ten times too large!

This may seem like a long journey through the drug disclosure label. However, this first experience is like getting a new computer. At first, it looks impossible. Then it seems difficult, but you make progress. Soon, much of the job will start to look easy. Remember that the drug label is not easy to read but is structured and written to draw your attention to the most important findings. For example, most of the time there will be a prominent warning—for the most serious cancer risks, for a drug with a tolerance problem, or for a very narrow indication.

A general word of caution about drug labels. Over thirty years' time, the FDA has consistently improved the completeness and uniformity of drug disclosure labels. (Unfortunately, they have not become more readable.) While new drug labels are much better than those of ten years ago, the older ones were not rewritten. (Nor, as noted earlier, have the older drugs been reevaluated for safety!) The older the drug, the less adequate will be the disclosure label. When a drug goes off patent and becomes generic, the labels are not updated as frequently. Also, the *Physicians' Desk Reference* does not contain the labels for many generic drugs. (That is a separate volume.) However, a large share of the most frequently prescribed drugs have adequate and up-to-date labels.

Finally, don't worry about ending up with more questions than answers. Reading a book chapter and a few drug labels is not enough background to make changes in your drug regimen by yourself. The idea is to get a sense of the real risks and benefits, and to generate some questions to take up with your pharmacist or doctor. As the next chapter will explain, talking to your doctor when you have questions about the prescription written is not always easy.

CHAPTER FOURTEEN

Talking to Your Doctor

THE WOMAN ON THE telephone had that slightly shrill edge to her voice that signals the beginning of hysteria. "First, you need to calm down," said Diane Rehm. "Just calm down." Rehm is the host of a popular Washington, D.C., radio talk show. I was the guest, and directly responsible for this caller's distress. The subject was Tambocor and similar drugs for irregular heartbeats. I was asking why 25 percent of doctors continued to prescribe these drugs for patients with mild irregular heartbeats despite clear, widely publicized scientific evidence that they could cause cardiac arrest. Both the woman on the telephone and her husband were taking these drugs. No wonder she was concerned.

After the distress level had dropped, I told the caller she needed to discuss this with her doctor. Then I gave the warning I always provide when so little information is available about someone's medical history and other medication. She shouldn't make any changes in her medication before consulting with a physician.

"I can tell you right now what's going to happen," the woman said, "I will go to the doctor and tell him what you said." There was a pause. "He's going to tell me you're full of bunk! Then what am I going to do?"

Her comment hit a nerve. Two years earlier, I had been in Seattle doing research on these very drugs. I was staying with a family I had known for many years. One night over dinner, my host asked me what drugs I was investigating. "Is this one of them?" he asked. He put a bottle of medicine in the center of the dining room table. It was quinidine—one of these potentially lethal drugs—he had a heart rhythm problem so mild he couldn't sense it at all. Years earlier, it had been identified in an experimental heart screening test that is not recommended medical practice today. Later, back home, I wrote him a very carefully worded letter that quoted the FDA's recommendation (don't use this drug in such patients) and cited the scientific evidence (it had no benefits and caused cardiac arrest). I suggested he take this letter to his doctor and ask whether it was worth continuing the medication. The doctor told him to keep taking quinidine. I never learned whether he said I was full of bunk.

We hope that the world of medicine includes thousands upon thousands of doctors who will not be as defensive as these two stories suggest. But expressing doubts about medication once a doctor has prescribed it can be a tricky business. This chapter outlines a strategy with a good chance of working. In a more perfect system, consumers would automatically get understandable information about the risks and benefits of drugs instead of having to study a lengthy and complex drug disclosure label. In a more perfect system, getting an independent evaluation of your medication would be as straightforward as requesting a second opinion before surgery.

The main idea is to use the features of the system that are likely to help you. For example, doctors are trained to listen carefully to their patients. It is a crucial part of reaching a successful diagnosis, and most doctors are good at it. Also, doctors are in a business, selling a service to the public. Like any business, they want as many satisfied customers are possible. An earlier chapter quoted the studies in which many doctors said they wrote some prescriptions because they thought patients wanted them, not because they would be effective. This is another indication of how carefully doctors listen to their patients. Some readers may know their doctors so well it's like talking to an old friend. But for most of us, a doctor's appointment is so structured that it is almost like playing a part in a brief movie script. The patient describes the problem and answers questions. The doctor conducts a examination. This results in a diagnosis and treatment, most often a prescription. The plan most likely to succeed is to work within one of the standard scripts that describe most meetings between doctor and patient.

Just as an earlier chapter suggested a balanced but skeptical attitude toward prescription drugs, a similarly moderate approach is also the best strategy for talking to your doctor. Extreme approaches can lead to problems. If you are afraid to ask any questions, it is going to be difficult to get involved in decisions about your medication. Doctors have some patients who just want to be told what to do; with such patients that's most likely what will happen. You have the legal and ethical right to be a full participant in any decisions regarding your medical care. But if you get too aggressive and belligerent about exercising this seldom-realized right, you are likely to antagonize your doctor, which will not promote a productive relationship. The most useful approach is to think of a relationship with a doctor as a partnership. Richard Riegelman, a doctor who is dean of the School of Public Health and Health Services at George Washington University, describes a useful approach. The patient would say to the doctor, in effect, "Deal me in! I want a seat at the table when medical decisions are made about me." Let's see how to strengthen your role in that partnership when it comes to the drugs prescribed for you.

The first step is to think briefly about the other person in the partnership, the doctor. Doctors treat all kinds of patients. They may have other doctors and pharmacists as patients—people whose knowledge and experience with prescription drugs may equal or exceed their own. They also are sure to have patients with a blind faith that pills will solve their problems. Such patients can be found at the pharmacy every day over at the display of ginseng root or buying a book about the melatonin miracle. Others have religious or ethical objections to taking drugs. Most doctors are skilled in handling the wide variety of patient attitudes. However, to make this partnership work, the essential first step is to tell the doctor exactly where you fall on this spectrum. Don't imagine that everyone is like you or that the doctor can read your mind. For the system to give you even some of what you want, it's up to you to express clearly your attitude and expectations. I'm hoping many readers will be pleasantly surprised at the doctor's response.

At your next doctor's appointment—ideally a physical exam or routine follow-up visit—take a minute to describe your attitude toward prescription drugs. This is a kind of formal declaration in your partnership with your doctor, so I would suggest you do so in a particular way. Say something like, "I would like to discuss my *patient preferences* about medication, and hope you will make a note of them in my *medical record*." This simple sentence contains two medical phrases that have very specific and important meanings in the specialized medical language that doctors speak to each other. Doctors assume they'll be making the medical decisions; that's why you are paying for their expertise and many years of training. However, almost all doctors understand and respect "patient preferences" whether reasonable or not. (In a hospital coronary care unit I once met a woman with heart problems who vowed that no surgical instrument was ever to touch her heart, which belonged solely to God. That was patient preference, although an unusual one.) Talking about "patient preferences" is also a chance to voice your opinion without threatening the doctor's traditional turf. The second key phrase, "medical record," also has a special meaning. Everything important about you and your case gets written down in your medical record or chart. It is a polite way of saying to your doctor, "Now this is important." This also has a great practical value. Doctors might see more than a hundred patients a week. They can't possibly remember every conversation with a patient. They refresh their memory by checking each patient's chart or medical record. Also, if you're in one of those group practices where you might see different doctors on different days, it is absolutely essential to have your preferences recorded on your medical record. Your record is how doctors and nurses communicate with each other about you.

Before you ask to have your patient preference noted in your medical record, it's up to you to decide what those preferences might be. Everyone is different. Personally, I would probably say something like this: "I would like to know as much as possible about the risks and benefits of any drugs you might prescribe. Please tell me about all the serious risks, even if they are rare. I'm interested in knowing the alternatives, too, including what would happen with no treatment."

However, I know people who are even more cautious about taking drugs than I am. One friend of mine might say, "I want to take as few drugs as possible. To avoid taking drugs I am even willing to suffer some discomfort." And of course I know many people who might say, "I'm willing to take any drug you think might have a chance of helping me." If this last statement describes your patient preference, I'm not sure it's worth going through this whole exercise, because that is what the doctor will probably assume unless you say otherwise. But if your own preference differs, you will benefit by expressing it to the doctor and asking that it be included in your medical record. This conversation about your preferences can be very brief; you can plan out ahead of time what you want to say. If you don't get a useful response, this is an important warning flag that you need to find a doctor with whom you can communicate more effectively.

The next step is to ask your doctor to review all the prescriptions you now take. Some people call it a "brown bag" session because you can put all your medication in a brown bag and take it to the doctor who provides your primary medical care. Then together you can review all the drugs prescribed by any doctor for any purpose. That is the easiest approach, and it can be combined with your discussion of preferences. However, your new partnership with your doctor will start on a better footing if you have completed some of the homework described in the previous chapters. You can take to a brown bag session your medication register and any questions from your review of the drug disclosure labels.

You can always ask certain standard questions about your medications. It's a good idea to bring these and your own questions in writing to the doctor's appointment.

1. Does my medical record reflect my drug allergies? Can I have a list of the drugs I need to avoid?
2. Can any of the drugs I'm taking be discontinued now? Which drugs can I discontinue myself and which drugs require your help?
3. Are there any drug interactions, or duplications of drugs to worry about?
4. Are there any alternatives available that are either safer or cheaper?
5. Do I have a condition for which a drug-free trial might

work? (Many people who have taken drugs for depression, high blood pressure, cholesterol, certain heart problems, or pain often find they can halt the drug. Some people taking drugs for high blood pressure or cholesterol discover the test results remain at or near normal without the drug.)

6. Am I due any laboratory tests to check for drug effects? (Try to get a schedule for any regular testing.)

7. Are there any signs or symptoms I should watch for, given my own particular mix of drugs?

You also may have generated some specific questions from your review of the drug disclosure labels. Once again, it is helpful to have them in writing. Also, you should be prepared for the fact that many doctors believe the drug labels are not helpful. They rarely consult the disclosure labels and may be entirely unaware of the interesting material you have discovered. Just as few doctors report adverse reactions directly to the FDA, only a small number appreciate the detail and accuracy of the information on the label. Also, like consumers, doctors find labels difficult to work with. So be prepared for a negative reaction to the drug disclosure labeling. But your questions are still good ones, and a competent doctor should respond to your concerns.

The first step, then, is to make sure the doctor understands your preferences and has them on record. The second is a medication review, or brown bag session. A third action you can take to play a role in decisions about medications is always appropriate: Bring any suspected adverse effects to the doctor's attention. A majority of the time, drugs should not produce continuing adverse effects. This is particularly true for the drugs people take for months or years on end, such as cholesterol- or blood-pressure-lowering drugs, pills for weight reduction, painkillers for arthritis, and medication for asthma.

Even with drugs with a high risk of adverse effects—such as drugs for depression—adjustment of dose and trials with a different medication ought to help keep unpleasant side effects to a minimum. Many people mistakenly believe they have to put up with annoying or unpleasant side effects. However, a patient needing help for side effects is a familiar problem that doctors are trained to handle. Put another way, if a drug is producing any suspected adverse effects, doctors will expect the patient to ask the doctor to review the prescribing decision for adjustments. If you are experiencing an adverse effect, be sure to bring in your medication register; don't just focus on the most recently prescribed drug. Once the door to discussing your medication is opened in this fashion, you can raise any other questions about this drug or others. Can you discontinue this medication? What are the alternatives?

These three strategies give the best chance for a productive discussion with your doctor about medication. Unfortunately, there are no guarantees of success. You can become a good partner in making medication decisions. But the doctor has to be a good partner too. So it is also worth thinking about some of the things doctors are likely to say—and not say—in response to your expressed concerns. It is inaccurate and unfair to talk about doctors as if they were all identical.

Some doctors have a heavy hand with the prescribing pen; they see a lot of patients and send most of them away with a prescription. (Identifying and cultivating heavy prescribers is a key task for a drug company sales force.) Other doctors—maybe not too many—are reluctant to prescribe drugs and will urge a serious trial of nondrug alternatives whenever possible. (A few M.D.'s favor natural and herbal remedies.) And most doctors fall somewhere in between. It is worth knowing whether you are dealing with a heavy prescriber, a sparing prescriber, or someone in between. Doctors who prescribe a lot of drugs may not announce their policy other than to hand you a sample of a new drug when the old drug was working fine. A patient (who can't observe a doctor every day) might notice that almost every appointment ends with a prescription—and often a free drug sample. Some offices are filled with posters, brochures, and other materials with a drug company logo, a sign that the drug company representatives are lavishing giveaways on this doctor. At the other end of the spectrum, doctors who are reluctant to prescribe drugs are more likely to tell you their policy. (This is probably because many doctors believe patients expect drugs as the easy solution, and they take extra time to explain their approach.) Possibly the best way to sense your own doctor's policy is to see how he or she responds to your concerns. There is no harm in asking your doctor to describe his or her own style of drug prescribing. Most doctors think they prescribe drugs "when they're needed" and may not know how they compare with other doctors.

As you get into a conversation about drugs with your doctor, you should keep something else in mind. For several reasons, many doctors are polished and skillfull in persuading patients to keep taking whatever drugs have already been prescribed. Doctors rightfully worry that patients won't take their prescribed medication. Part of this concern is based on clinical experience and medical research cited in an earlier chapter. As noted, a surprising number of patients don't take medication as prescribed. So when doctors start getting questions about the need for drugs, they begin to worry that the patient is not going to take them. Critical questions about drugs sometimes trigger a defensive response at a deeper and possibly unconscious level. Doctors are there to offer patients solutions to their medical problems. While a few medical specialties—notably surgery—focus on nondrug interventions, a prescription drug is the medical treatment that most doctors provide to a majority of their patients. When a skeptical patient starts questioning the need for prescription drugs, that patient is at some level expressing doubts about the main product that doctors have to offer.

These two factors explain why doctors often exaggerate the benefits of drugs and downplay the risks. They believe in the main health product they offer patients. The product can't help if the patients don't take the prescribed drug. So if you start asking questions about the drugs, don't be surprised to hear some scary talk designed to encourage you to keep taking your medication. Patients who initiate a discussion about the risks and benefits of the drugs the doctor has already prescribed need to be prepared for a strong argument why they should take them. Listen carefully, but don't forget you're the boss. In fact, one way you can evaluate the doctor is to gauge the extent to which he or she is responding to your concerns—or almost by reflex trying to make you a "compliant" patient. In truth, there is a kind of fear war going on. Some doctors are sure to criticize this book, charging that it is going to make patients afraid to take their needed medication. Many of these same doctors are then going to use fear to induce their patients to take drugs. They will say, "Your high blood pressure means that you could have a stroke! It's important to take the medication." (Very few will acknowledge that drug treatment for mild high blood pressure prevents strokes in only about 2 out of 1,000 patients who take the drug for a year, and about 3 will have a stroke anyway.)

Don't expect to hear prescribing errors openly admitted, despite the frightening statistics in the earlier chapter about physician prescribing errors. Many doctors are hesitant to tell patients about prescribing errors, even when they were made by other doctors. However, that doesn't mean that doctors won't correct a prescribing error if they observe one while reviewing your medication. Doctors who really think, "Why on earth is this patient on this medication?" are more likely to say something like, "Let's see how well you do without this drug." Or else they might say, "I have a newer, better, safer drug I'd like you to try." If a review of your medication discloses some serious mistakes, don't expect to hear about it. Although I know doctors who are very direct and very frank about medical errors, a more likely outcome is that medication adjustments will be made with a silken smooth explanation intended to provoke neither patient fears nor unwanted patient curiosity.

In sizing up your doctor's response, it is important not to confuse a friendly bedside manner with a genuine response to your concerns. Because of their unique role, job pressures, and intense training, doctors are in some ways quite similar. They perform one of those special jobs—like police officers—that seem to mold the person. A varied style in dealing with patients tends to be the exception to the many similar traits that a majority of doctors share. Some very good doctors have a cold, brusque manner. Others may have an open, friendly, and reassuring manner but make frequent mistakes. Also, there are doctors (often the older ones) who believe patients want them to make all the decisions. There are doctors (often the younger ones) who actively seek patient participation in medical decision making and who welcome questions and expect to adapt to patient preferences.

After approaching the doctor with one of the strategies described above, it is time to remember you're still the boss. It's up to you to think about your original concerns and decide how the doctor handled them. With a drug register, some homework on the drugs you're taking, and one of these strategies, we can hope you will get a result that will satisfy you. It is also possible you will be unhappy with the outcome. Or possibly you've already had other concerns about this doctor. If you are not satisfied, it may be time to ask another doctor to take a fresh look at your health and medication. You may not necessarily want to switch doctors, but you have some concerns. Let's examine what to do next.

With a traditional diagnosis—for example, a recommendation for surgery—the standard solution is to get a second opinion. For the most expensive procedures, insurance and managed care companies often require one. Unfortunately, seeking a second opinion on one or more prescriptions is a little more unusual. However, it is the theme of this chapter that most patients will get the best results by asking for a service the system is accustomed to providing routinely, thus playing a part in one of the prepared scripts. So if you decide that you are not satisfied with your doctor, one solution is to shop for a new one. Following a few rules will increase your chances of success. This is how I suggest looking for a new doctor, and testing how the doctor responds to your concerns.

If all you are seeking is a chance to talk to another doctor about your medication, then all you need to ask for is a consultation. This would typically result in a single appointment of about fifteen minutes in which you could go over your medication and your questions. If you're seriously looking for another doctor, you also might want to begin a potential new relationship by getting a full-fledged physical exam. (Depending on your medical care plan, it may also be more expensive.) With more information about your medical history, you are likely to get better answers to your questions. As it happens, a physical is a very standard first medical service that primary care doctors regularly provide. Doctors also like to acquire new patients, and a physical is the usual starting point. So that's how you can get a new doctor to take a fresh look at your medication; you get a physical exam and a new perspective on your overall situation in the bargain. The next problem is finding the right doctor.

First, ask your friends what they think of their doctors. Often, patients really like the best doctors. Word gets around. But remember, you're looking for a doctor who is comfortable with questions from patients. So a friend who loves her doctor but just wants to be told what to do may not be a good source for a recommendation. An acquaintance who is a nurse or other medical professional can often help. Word of mouth or asking in some community group where you already belong often produces a list of candidates. If it doesn't, the next stop is a doctor referral service at one of the local hospitals. Doctors are vital customers for hospitals. It is the doctors who send the hospitals the patients. And without enough patients, hospitals have to close their doors. One of the many perks hospitals use to woo doctors is a referral service for new patients. (Usually a welcome sight in a doctor's office.) To do business with a particular hospital, doctors have to be granted privileges by a committee that inspects their background and credentials. The best hospital in town is likely (no guarantees here) to have attracted the best doctors and asked the most questions about their background and experience. However, you can consider other factors. If you want a doctor's office reasonably near your home, contact the nearest hospital. Usually, doctors like to have offices near the hospital where most of their patients are being treated. When you call a hospital referral service, don't expect to hear any opinions about what the doctors are like. But the service will provide a few details such as the doctor's sex, age, medical school, residency, and qualifications. The truth is that it is very hard to find out anything useful about doctors from almost any source. A referral service will provide some basic facts if your own network of friends and contacts doesn't produce a more likely candidate.

When you have selected a name, make an appointment. Say you are a new patient, and ask to schedule a consultation or a physical exam. One word of warning. If you are looking for a fresh opinion, don't go to a doctor in the same office or medical group as the one you now have. You are likely to find too many similarities and get questions about why you're not seeing your usual doctor. Some HMOs and managed care plans limit the doctors you can see, but often make it easier to switch. Some plans even advertise that you can "pick" your doctor, and set up a system to make the choices easier.

Your first appointment is the perfect time to discuss your patient preferences, bring in your medication register, and talk about any adverse effects. Because you are building a new relationship, seeing a new doctor is a little like dating. When you go out with someone new, the focus is not likely to be on what happened with your previous boyfriend or girlfriend. So there is little benefit in dwelling on problems with your previous doctor unless you have specific medical issues the new doctor needs to address. Another way to answer questions about why you are changing doctors is to put your desires in a positive light: "I'm looking for a doctor who can take a little more time to talk to me when medication is prescribed." Focus on seeing whether you can build a working partnership with this doctor. Getting the physical exam does not irrevocably commit you to continuing with the new doctor. After the first appointment, you might be asked to schedule a follow-up appointment—perhaps to check the effects of a medication adjustment. If you decide against the new doctor, you can always cancel the second appointment by telephone.

You're the boss, and only you can choose your doctor. You're the boss, and with a doctor's help, only you can decide which medications you want to take over the long term. While there is no such thing as a safe drug, many drugs provide tremendous benefits that greatly outweigh their risks. On the other hand, many people are taking medication that provides little benefit, that they should have stopped months ago, or that is doing more harm than good. Ultimately, the choice to take medicine, and which medicine, is up to you. You're the boss, but don't forget to follow the instructions. Those pills nestled in the bottom of the medicine bottle only look simple. They are in fact some of the most complex and powerful biological tools ever conceived by science. You must use them wisely. Our whole society needs to learn how to use prescription drugs more safely. These last three chapters described the steps you can take yourself. The rest we'll have to do together. Change will begin to happen when people like you start to demand it.

ACKNOWLEDGMENTS

ANY BOOK WITH references to so many scientific studies ought to hint at the burden of scholarship and research involved. As the research assistant for this book, Jock Friedly made invaluable contributions through his skill in tracking down the complete scientific record on a very large variety of topics from many different kinds of sources. Whether it was the yellowed pages of congressional hearings held decades ago, out-of-print reports, or obscure scientific journals, he could find them. His understanding of the subject and his initiative often opened whole new avenues of research.

In a book of this technical complexity, the author alone remains responsible for the scientific and medical accuracy. However, I could not have attempted this task without the assistance of many expert reviewers and advisors. Throughout the writing of this book, Curt Furberg M.D., Ph.D., and Bruce Psaty, M.D., Ph.D., were kind enough to review chapters and drafts and provide many helpful comments. Sidney Wolfe, M.D., provided many helpful suggestions and generously shared the research files of the Public Citizen Health Research Group. In addition, I am indebted to Peter Breggin, M.D., for reviewing the manuscript for references to psychoactive drugs and for generously sharing his voluminous research files on that subject. Steven Baskin, Ph.D., provided me with invaluable help on toxicology. Larry Sasich, Pharm.D., provided many valuable documents and his own insights on two important issues: consumer information and labeling, and pharmacy. Raymond Woosley, M.D., Ph.D., provided many helpful suggestions and references about the properties of nonsedating antihistamines. Richard Riegelman, M.D., M.P.H., provided helpful comments about the content of the opening chapter. Bradford C. Roberts made helpful suggestions and comments for the chapters explaining what consumers can do. Milton Carrow, J.D., provided comments over many months, helping me to see this issue from the perspective of the informed reader. However, in listing the names of the people who so generously assisted me, I am not implying that they endorse my own views or interpretation of the facts.

The Food and Drug Administration deserves special thanks for providing information, including hundreds of documents about its activities. I continue to believe that the FDA has one of the best records in government in providing information to the public. The Freedom of Information Staff and the Division of Pharmacovigilance and Epidemiology spent many hours responding to my requests. I appreciate the extra efforts of Donald McClearn in the Office of Public Affairs, Robert Temple, M.D., in the Center for Drug Evaluation and Research, and Betty Dorsey of the Freedom of Information Staff.

At George Washington University, the Center for Health Policy Research continued to provide a stimulating and hospitable environment for research and writing. I am grateful to the director, Sara Rosenbaum, for her support. Also, without the administrative help of Ali Naderzad and Helen Naumah, my life would have been difficult indeed.

I am particularly indebted to Bob Bender, my editor at Simon & Schuster. His interest and belief in this book played a key role throughout its long journey from the germ of an idea to a finished book on the shelves. At International Creative Management, my agent Esther Newberg continued to provide her able representation and support.

Finally, I would like to thank my wife, Barbara, not only for many valuable comments and editorial suggestions, but for her love, support, and patience during a long and difficult project.

NOTES

THROUGHOUT THE BOOK, I have sought to document the findings in accepted scholarly form. However, a few special rules do apply to the many endnotes.

The product disclosure statement, drug label, or package insert is the most authoritative and legally binding statements of the known properties of a prescription drug. These disclosure statements come from the manufacturer but are periodically reviewed for accuracy and completeness by the FDA staff. Throughout the book, the disclosure statements are used as a principal source to document the properties of drugs. Most but not all of these statements are collected in a commercial book called the *Physicians' Desk Reference*, published annually. When I cite a property of a drug in this book, the footnote simply says "*Physicians' Desk Reference*." To find the information, simply look up the chemical or brand name of the drug in the current year's volume. Page numbers are not included since they are different in each year's edition. The same information is included on the fine-print leaflet called the package insert. It can be obtained at the pharmacy. Disclosure statements change frequently, but the changes tend to be minor, and it is rare for warnings or adverse effects to disappear from the label. New cautions and new medical uses of drugs do appear.

The second benchmark source for the properties of prescription drugs is in the pharmacology text *Goodman and Gilman's The Pharmacological Basis of Therapeutics*, 1996 edition. It is an extensive volume and widely available in libraries. When the properties of drugs are cited in this volume, the reference will read "Goodman and Gilman" and the page numbers.

Two often-cited medical journals have changed their names recently. *The Journal of the American Medical Association* has become *JAMA*, which is what everybody called it anyway. All citations are for the abbreviated name. Similarly, the *British Medical Journal* has become *BMJ*.

Finally, the patient names are real names, except I used a pseudonym for those who requested it and for Internet newsgroup postings unless the person involved consented. The names in this book that are pseudonyms are: Glenn St. John, James Smith, Sara Huxford, James Morton, Barbara Wilkes, Michael Sharkey, and William Corson. Cases taken from medical journals are identified exactly as they appeared in the original publication.

1. WARNING FLAGS

1. Affidavit of Joseph Burton, pathologist, in *Kaufman v. Janssen Pharmaceutica*, Fulton County, Georgia, 95-VS-95077-E. Janssen paid Kaufman damages in the case, but the amount is under seal.
2. *Physicians' Desk Reference*.
3. U.S. Department of Health and Human Services, Food and Drug Administration, "Terfenadine: Proposal to Withdraw Ap-

proval of Two New Drug Applications and One Abbreviated New Drug Application," *Federal Register,* January 14, 1997, pp. 1889–92.

4. U.S. Department of Health and Human Services, Food and Drug Administration, Spontaneous Reported System, Division of Epidemiology and Surveillance, as of May 19, 1994.

5. U.S. Department of Health and Human Services, Food and Drug Administration, "Guideline for Postmarketing Reporting of Adverse Drug Experiences," Docket no. 85D-0249, Market 1992. The only requirement of federal law is that if a manufacturer learns of a possible drug-related death, it must forward this information to the FDA.

6. R. N. Anderson et al., "Final Report of Final Mortality Statistics, 1995," *Monthly Vital Statistics Report 45,* no. 11 (June 12, 1997). It includes certificates for Americans who die abroad. Table 10, page 40.

7. David A. Kessler, "Introducing MedWatch," *JAMA* 269 (1993):2765–67.

8. Estimates of severe injury and death are examined in chap. 3.

9. See chap. 8 for details.

10. J. L. Halaas et al., "Weight-Reducing Effects of the Plasma Protein Encoded by the Obese Gene," *Science* 269 (1995):543–46.

11. Boyce Rensberger, "Fabulous Discovery," *Washington Post,* July 27, 1995.

12. B. S. Hamilton et al., "Increased Obese mRNA Expression in Omental Fat Cells from Massively Obese Humans," *Nature Medicine)* 1 (1995):953–96.

13. This was a news group on the Internet: alt.support.prozac.survivors.

14. Peter D. Kramer, *Listening to Prozac* (New York: Viking Press, 1993), p.xv; IMS America, "Top 10 Products—United States: Total Sales Dollars," in *IMS America, Ltd.—Retail & Provider Perspective, 1997.* Reported $1.6 billion for Prozac in 1996.

15. Kramer, *Listening to Prozac,* pp. 12, 63, 64.

16. U.S. Department of Health and Human Services, Food and Drug Administration, Division of Drug Advertising, Marketing and Communications, letter to Eli Lilly, March 27, 1995.

17. Department of Health and Human Services, Food and Drug Administration, Division of Pharmacovigilance and Epidemiology, Spontaneous Reporting System. Calculated for the author for 1987 to 1997 as of July, 1997.

18. The chemically related Paxil and Zoloft caused a similar or larger number of adverse reactions in randomized clinical trials. But because sales are smaller than best-seller Prozac, and the drugs were on the market for fewer years, a smaller number of adverse reactions were reported to the FDA.

19. In my supermarket, the rat poison contained a close relative of warfarin, brodifacoum 3-[3-(3-4'-bromo-{1,1'-biphenyl}-4-yl)-1,2,3,4-tetrahydro-1-naphthalenyl\-4-hydroxy-2H-1-benzopyran-2-one.

20. Cheryl R. Nelson, "Drug Utilization in Office Practice," *Advance Data from Vital and Health Statistics of the Centers for Disease Control and Prevention*, no. 232, March 25, 1993, National Center for Health Statistics.

21. *Physicians' Desk Reference.*

22. *Drug Facts and Comparisons*, 1994 ed. (St. Louis: Facts & Comparisons, 1994), p. 2987.

23. Ibid. Curare preparations are Tubocuraine, metocuraine, p. 1533.

24. For an example, see "Kolyum Liquid" in the *Physicians' Desk Reference.*

25. Goodman and Gilman, pp. 219–21, 338.

26. William E. Pelham et al., "Separate and Combined Effects of Methylphenidate and Behavior Medication on Boys with Attention-Deficit Hyperactivity Disorder in the Classroom," *Journal of Consulting and Clinical Psychology* 61 (1993):506–15; Mark D. Rapoport et al., "Attention Deficit Disorder and Methylphenidate: Normalization Rates, Clinical Effectiveness, and Response Prediction in 76 Children," *Journal of the*

American Academy of Child and Adolescent Psychiatry 33 (1994):882–93.

27. V. I. Douglas, "Short-Term Effects of Methylphenidate on the Cognitive, Learning, and Academic Performance of Children with Attention Deficit Disorder in the Laboratory and the Classroom," *Journal of Child Psychology and Psychiatry* 27 (1986):191–211.

28. Judith L. Rapoport et al., "Dextroamphetamine: Cognitive and Behavorial Effects in Normal Prepubertal Boys," *Science* 199 (1978):560–62.

29. Benjamin L. Handen et al., "Adverse Side Effects of Methylphenidate Among Mentally Retarded Children with ADHD," *Journal of the American Academy of Child and Adolescent Psychiatry* 30, no.2 (1991):241–45. Although mainly focusing on adverse effects, the authors sum up: "While there is growing evidence that mentally retarded children respond to stimulant medication with rates similar to non-retarded peers, this population may be at greater risk for developing motor tics and becoming socially withdrawn."

30. American Psychiatric Association, *Diagnostic and Statistical Manual of Mental Disorders* (DSM-IV) (Washington, D.C.: American Psychiatric Association, 1994), pp. 78–85.

31. *Physicians' Desk Reference.* As the manufacturer sums up, "The specific [cause] is unknown."

32. *Physicians' Desk Reference.*

33. D. J. Safer et al., "Increased Methylphenidate Usage for Attention Deficit Disorder in the 1990s," *Pediatrics* 98 (1996):1084–88.

34. W. A. Ray et al., "A Study of Anti-Psychotic Drug Use in Nursing Homes: Epidemiologic Evidence Suggesting Misuse," *American Journal of Public Health* 70 (1980):485–91. Psychotropic drugs are given almost universally to the inmates of psychiatric facilities, often without their consent. A study of 173 Tennessee nursing homes showed 43 percent of patients receiving psychotropic drugs, a condition the authors described as "misuse."

35. *Physicians' Desk Reference.*

36. Paul H. Lipkin et al., "Tics and Dyskinesia Associated with Stimulant Treatment in Attention-Deficit Hyperactivity Disorder," *Archives of Pediatrics & Adolescent Medicine* 148 (1994):859–61.

37. Breck G. Bocherding et al., "Motor/Vocal Tics and Compulsive Behaviors on Stimulant Drugs: Is There a Common Vulnerability?" *Psychiatry Research* 33 (1990):83–94.

38. Russell A. Barkley, "Side Effects of Methylphenidate in Children with Attention Deficit Hyperactivity Disorder: A Systemic, Placebo-Controlled Evaluation," *Pediatrics* 86 (1990):184–92. To avoid exaggeration, the side effects reported by those on the drug were subtracted from the number of similar effects of those on a placebo. Data calculated from table 3.

39. *Physicians' Desk Reference.*

40. James H. Satterfield, "Growth of Hyperactive Children Treated with Methylphenidate," *Archives of General Psychiatry* 36 (1979):212–17.

41. *Physicians' Desk Reference.*

42. Russell A. Barkley, *Attention-Deficit Hyperactivity Disorder* (New York: Guilford Press, 1990), p. 581.

43. Ibid., p. 589.

44. Search "methylphenidate" on the Drug Enforcement Administration's Internet Web site to see their current thinking.

45. Thomas J. Moore, *Deadly Medicine: Why Tens of Thousands of Heart Patients Died in America's Worse Drug Disaster* (New York: Simon & Schuster, 1995).

46. Business Watch, Exhibit 3, "Dollar Sales Volume," *Medical Marketing and Media,* April 1995, pp. 66–76.

47. Sprint Study Group, "The Secondary Prevention Re-Infarction Israeli Nifedipine Trial (SPRINT) II: Results," *European Heart Journal* 9 (1988):(suppl)350A; Uri Elkayam, et al., "A Prospective, Randomized, Double-Blind, Crossover Study to Compare the Efficacy and Safety of Chronic Nifedipine Therapy with That of Isosorbide Dinitrate," *Circulation* 82 (1990):1954–61; R. J. Wilcox et al., "Trial of Early Nifedipine in

Acute Myocardial Infarction: The Trent Study," *BMJ* 293 (1986): 1204–8; P. R. Licthlen et al., "Retardation of Angiographic Progression of Coronary Artery Disease by Nifedipine," *Lancet* 335 (1990):1109–19. The authors claim a tiny effect in fewer new lesions in the arteries. Other observers noted the excess deaths among those treated with the active drug (8 deaths in treatment group vs. 2 in placebo group); B. M. Psaty et al., "The Risk of Myocardial Infarction Associated with Antihypertensive Drug Therapies," *JAMA* 274 (1995):620–25; M. Pahor et al., "Long-Term Survival and Use of Antihypertensive Medications in Older Persons," *Journal of the American Geriatric Society* 43 (1995):1191–97; Holland Interuniversity Nifedipine/Metroprolol Trial (HINT) Research Group, "Early Treatment of Unstable Angina in the Coronary Care Unit," *British Heart Journal* 56 (1985):400–413.

48. Psaty, "The Risk of Myocardial Infarction."

49. Curt F. Furberg, personal communication. A trial of nimodipine to reduce cerebrovascular complications of heart valve replacement surgery was halted after eight patients died in treatment group, compared to one on placebo.

50. Marco Pahor et al., "Do Calcium Channel Blockers Increase the Risk of Cancer?" *American Journal of Hypertension* 9 (1996):695–99. Marco Pahor et al., "Calcium Channel Blockade and Incidence of Cancer in Aged Populations," *Lancet* 348 (1996):493–97.

51. J. E. Buring et al., "Calcium Channel Blockers and Myocardial Infarction: A Hypothesis Formulated but Not Yet Tested," *JAMA* 274 (1995):654–55; Lionel H. Opie and Frank H. Messerli, "Nifedipine and Mortality: Grave Defects in the Dossier," *Circulation* 92 (1995):1068–73; Robert A. Kloner, "Nifedipine in Ischemic Heart Disease," *Circulation* 92(1995): 1074–77.

52. American College of Cardiology, "Joint ACC/AMA Statement on the Psaty Study Regarding Calcium Channel Blockers," press release, March 19, 1995.

53. Pfizer Inc. advertisement in *New England Journal of Medicine* (1996).

54. E. Grossman and Frank H. Messerli, "Calcium Antagonists in Cardiovascular Disease: A Necessary Controversy But an Unnecessary Panic," *American Journal of Medicine* 102(1997):147–49.

55. Lauren B. Leveton et al., eds., *HIV and the Blood Supply: An Analysis of Crisis Decisionmaking,* Institute of Medicine (Washington D.C.: National Academy Press, 1995). Appendix D.

56. See chap. 10, "The Doctor's Office."

2. DRUG SAFETY

1. Scandinavian Simvastatin Survival Study Group, "Randomized Trial of Cholesterol Lowering in 444 Patients with Coronary Heart Disease: The Scandinavian Simvastatin Survival Study (4S)," *Lancet* 334 (1994):1383–89.

2. IMS America, "Leading 50 Drugs in 1995 by Total Rx," press release.

3. C. D. Klaassen, ed., *Casarett & Doull's Toxicology: The Basic Science of Poisons* (New York: McGraw-Hill, 1996). See chap. 8, "Chemical Carcinogenesis."

4. The drug disclosure labels of these drugs do not contain any statements about cancer testing.

5. Once again, the drug disclosure label is used as the authoritative listing of adverse effects. Others may appear in scientific literature but are denied by the manufacturer.

6. Goodman and Gilman, p. 1086. It is amazing that the incidence of the most common and potentially dangerous allergic reaction in pharmacology cannot be pinpointed with greater precision than from 0.7 percent to 11 percent. The midpoint of that ranges appears in the text.

7. As noted in the previous chapter, the FDA sought to withdraw Seldane because of the danger of its producing cardiac effects.

8. See chap. 8.

9. See chap. 6.

10. Some molecules come in mirror-image shapes (something

like looking at the letter *y* in a mirror) called isomers. Synthroid is the *l* isomer, and the thyroid hormone used to lower cholesterol levels is the *d* isomer. Some drugs also come in mixtures containing both isomers.

11. Coronary Drug Project Research Group, "The Coronary Drug Project: Findings Leading to Further Modifications of Its Protocol with Respect to Dextrothyroxine," *JAMA* 220 (1972):996–1008.

12. Dehydroepiandrosterone, or DHEA, is a human hormone of unknown function that has become popular as an "antiaging" compound because DHEA levels peak at age twenty-five and decline in inverse proportion to the aging process. Thomas J. Moore, *Lifespan: Who Lives Longer and Why* (New York: Simon & Schuster, 1993), pp. 260–62.

13. M. L. Kamb et al., "Eosinophilia-Myalgia Syndrome in L-Tryptophan-Exposed Patients," *JAMA* 267 (1992):77–82.

14. G. S. Omenn et al., "Effects of a Combination of Beta Carotene and Vitamin A on Lung Cancer and Cardiovascular Disease," *New England Journal of Medicine* 334 (1996):1150–55.

15. Moore, *Lifespan*, pp. 260–62.

16. R. P. Ahlquist, "A Study of the Adrenotropic Receptors," *American Journal of Physiology* 153 (1948):586–600.

17. M. Weatherall, *In Search of a Cure: A History of Pharmaceutical Discovery* (Oxford: Oxford University Press, 1990), pp. 240–42; W. Koberstein and S. Schuber, "Sir James Black: Executive Profile," *Pharmaceutical Executive*, February 1989, pp. 30–42.

18. These adverse effects were listed by the manufacturer in the drug disclosure labels and captured by a computer search of the texts, published as the CD-ROM version of the *Physicians' Desk Reference*.

19. Goodman and Gilman, p. 150.

3. THE DANGERS OF DRUGS

1. Thomas J. Moore, *Deadly Medicine* (New York: Simon & Schuster, 1995).

2. Ibid. The appendix calculations suggest that these drugs caused from 26,000 to 66,000 deaths annually during the year of highest prescription volume. All but one of the drugs are still approved and marketed and continue to cause thousands of deaths each year.

3. What doctors tell patients about the risks of drugs is described in detail in chap. 10.

4. U.S. Department of Commerce, Bureau of the Census, *Statistical Abstracts of the United States,* 1995 (Washington, D.C.: Government Printing Office, 1996), table 678.

5. Ibid., table 134.

6. E.g., allergic reactions—penicillin; heart rhythym disruptions—Lanoxin; agranulocytosis—Procainamide; bizarre behavior—Prozac; liver damage—halothane; gallstones—Lopid; internal bleeding—nonsteroidal anti-inflammatory drugs.

7. J. W. Smith et al., "Studies on the Epidemiology of Adverse Reactions," *Annals of Internal Medicine* 65 (1966):629–40.

8. R. I. Ogilvie and J. Ruedy, "Adverse Reactions During Hospitalization," *Canadian Medical Association Journal* 97 (1967):1450–57.

9. P. Gardner and L. J. Watson, "Adverse Reactions: A Pharmacist-Based Monitoring System," *Clinical Pharmacology and Therapeutics* 11 (1970):802–7.

10. P. A. Frisk et al., "Community-Hospital Pharmacist Detection of Drug-Related Problems upon Patient Admission to Small Hospitals," *American Journal of Hospital Pharmacy* 37 (1977): 738–42.

11. A. A. Mitchell et al., "Adverse Reactions in Children Leading to Hospital Admission," *Pediatrics* 82 (1988):24–29.

12. Ibid.

13. Thomas R. Einarson, "Drug-Related Hospital Admissions," *Annals of Pharmacotherapy* 27 (1993):832–39.

14. W. A. Ray et al., "Adverse Drug Reactions and the Elderly," *Health Affairs,* Fall 1990, pp. 114–22.

15. David Kessler et al., "Introducing MedWatch: A New Ap-

proach to Reporting Medication and Device Adverse Effects and Product Problems," *JAMA* 269 (1993):2765–68.

16. J. A. Johnson, and J. Lyle Bootman, 'Drug-Related Morbidity and Mortality," *Archives of Internal Medicine* 155 (1995):1949–56.

17. U.S. Department of Health and Human Services, National Center for Health Statistics, "Detailed Diagnoses and Procedures," *National Hospital Discharge Survey,* 1992. Calculated from 30.9 million hospital discharges. Despite major changes in population and aging, the hospitalization rate has changed little in twenty years.

18. From Einarson, "Drug-Related Hospital Admissions," and *National Hospital Discharge Survey.*

19. Pharmaceutical Research and Manufacturers of America, *PhRMA Facts & Figures Backgrounders: Drug Safety,* on the Internet at http://www.phrma.org/facts/bkgrndr/safety.html.

20. U.S. Department of Transportation, National Highway Traffic Safety Administration, *National Accident Sampling System/Crashworthiness Data System, 1991–1993,* report, p. 24. Includes injuries classified as serious, severe, critical, or maximum.

21. Calculated by the standard risk-assessment formula: (annual events x 70) / population.

22. D. W. Bates et al., "Incidence of Adverse Drug Events and Potential Adverse Drug Events: Implications for Prevention," *Jama* 274 (1995):29–34.

23. Ibid.

24. U.S. Bureau of the Census, *Statistical Abstracts of the United States,* 1992 (Washington, D.C.: Government Printing Office, 1993), calculated for 1990 from table 171.

25. American Hospital Association, *Hospital Statistics: The AHA Profile of United States Hospitals* (Chicago: American Hospital Association, 1994), p. xxxviii. Critics might argue in either direction whether these two famed institutions represent the typical community hospital. On one hand, a teaching hospital is likely to be referred the most serious and difficult cases. On the other,

these hospitals are reputed to attract the best and brightest in American medicine.

26. T. A. Brennan et al., "Incidence of Adverse Events and Negligence in Hospitalized Patients: Results of the Harvard Medical Practice Study," *New England Journal of Medicine* 324 (1991):370–84.

27. D. C. Classen et al., "Adverse Drug Events in Hospitalized Patients," *JAMA* 277 (1997):301–6; R. B. Talley, "Drug-Induced Illness," *JAMA* 229 (1974):1043.

28. U.S. Bureau of the Census, *Statistical Abstracts of the United States,* 1995 data for 1993 rounded to the nearest thousand. From table 131 except motor vehicle, table 129, and commercial air, table 989. On-the-job accidents are reduced downward from the published total to prevent double counting with homicide (1,024 on the job) and motor vehicle (1,329). Drug-death estimates are my own.

29. U.S. Department of Health and Human Services, National Center for Health Statistics, *Vital Statistics of the United States,* vol. 2, *Mortality,* pt. A (Washington, D.C.: Public Health Service, 1996).

30. J. S. Swann et al., *Annual Adverse Drug Experience Report, 1991* (Washington, D.C.: Food and Drug Administration, n.d.).

31. National Cancer Institute et al., *DES Basic Booklet* (National DES Educational Program, 1992).

32. U.S. Department of Health and Human Services, Food and Drug Administration, "Phenformin," *FDA Drug Bulletin,* August 1977, pp. 14–16. This report estimated approximately 2 cases per 1,000 patients and 380,000 patients on the drug.

33. Goodman and Gilman, p. 414.

34. Peter R. Breggin, *Brain-Disabling Treatments in Psychiatry* (New York: Spring-Verlag, 1997), chap. 3.

35. Ibid.

36. Goodman and Gilman, p. 416; Peter R. Breggin, *Toxic Psychiatry* (New York: St Martin's Press, 1991), pp. 74–75.

37. J. M. Kane, "Schizophrenia," *New England Journal of Medicine* 334 (1996):34–41.

38. Goodman and Gilman, p. 414.

4. THE BENEFITS OF DRUGS

1. James B. Wyngaarden and Lloyd H. Smith, Jr., eds., *Cecil Textbook of Medicine* 19th ed. (Philadelphia: W. B. Saunders Co., 1992), p. 1292. A prevalence of 0.2 to 0.3 percent.

2. United States Pharmacopeia, 1996, personal communication. There were 3,291 FDA-approved drugs for which full chemical descriptions of strength and purity had been compiled and published as of May 16, 1996. Drugs that sold in two forms—for example as a pill and as ointment—are counted separately.

3. Medical Research Council Working Party, "MRC Trial of Treatment of Mild Hypertension: Principal Results," *BMJ* 291 (1985):97–104.

4. K. L. Davis et al., "A Double-Blind Placebo-Controlled Multicenter Study of Tacrine for Alzheimer's Disease," *New England Journal of Medicine* 327 (1992):1253–59.

5. Rate quoted by CVS drugstores in Washington, D.C., on June 10, 1996, for 20 mg q.i.d.: $137 a month.

6. Davis et al., "A Double-Blind . . . Study." Substantial liver damage is defined here as serum alanine aminotranferase values three times the upper limit of normal.

7. Joseph A. DiMasi, "Success Rates for New Drugs Entering Clinical Testing in the United States," *Clinical Pharmacology and Therapeutics* 58 (1995):1–14. Among the 90 percent of drugs that fail to reach the market after starting human testing, 46 percent are abandoned because of problems with efficacy, compared to 27 percent for safety.

8. Norman Cousins, *Head First: The Biology of Hope* (New York: E. P. Dutton, 1989).

9. Andrew Weil, *Spontaneous Healing* (New York: Fawcett Columbine, 1995), pp. 55–58.

10. Caryle Hirschberg and Marc Ian Barasch, *Remarkable Recovery: What Extraordinary Healings Tell Us About Getting Well and Staying Well* (New York: Riverhead Books, 1995), pp. 37–38.

11. Ibid. They in fact argue that there may be more cases than one-per-doctor-per-lifetime. But perhaps not many more cases.

12. Leonard Cobb, "A Sham Operation . . ." *New England Journal of Medicine* 250 (1959):114–17.

13. Howard Brody, "The Lie That Heals: The Ethics of Giving Placebos," *Annals of Internal Medicine* 97 (1982):112–18.

14. "Smithkline Beecham Paxil Eliminates Full Panic Attacks in 76%," *The Pink Sheet*, May 13, 1996, pp. T, G 2.

15. R. A. Barkley, *Attention Deficit Hyperactivity Disorder* (New York: Guilford Press, 1990), p. 577.

16. Joan-Ramon Laporte and Albert Figueras, "Placebo Effects in Psychiatry," *Lancet* 334 (1993):1206–8.

17. Management Committee, "The Australian Therapeutic Trial in Mild Hypertension," *Lancet* (14 June 1980) pp. 1261–67.

18. J. L. Anderson, "Relationship of Baseline Characteristics to Suppression of Ventricular Arrhythmias During Placebo and Active Therapy in Patients After Myocardial Infarction," *Circulation* 79 (1989):610–19.

19. Milton Packer, "The Placebo Effect in Heart Failure," *American Heart Journal* 120 (1990):1579–82.

20. Goodman and Gilman, p. 438.

21. J. F. Wernicke et al., "Fixed Dose Fluoxetine Therapy for Depression," *Psychopharmacology Bulletin* 23 (1987):164–68.

22. American Psychiatric Association, *Diagnostic and Statistical Manual of Mental Disorders,* 4th ed. (DSM-IV) (Washington D.C.: American Psychiatric Association, 1994). This document provides the "official list" of symptoms for the various psychiatric disorders, including depression.

23. W. F. Byerly et al., "Fluoxetine, a Selective Serotonin Uptake Inhibitor, for the Treatment of Outpatients with Major Depression," *Journal of Clinical Psychopharmacology* 8 (1988):112–15.

24. U.S. Department of Health and Human Services, Food and Drug Administration, "Review and Evaluation of Clinical Data: Nefazodone," September 15, 1992. In this review of Serzone (ne-

fazodone), Bristol-Meyers failed to demonstrate efficacy in six of eight clinical trials.

25. R. W. Sherwin, "Serum Cholesterol Levels and Cancer Mortality in 361,662 Men Screened for the Multiple Risk Factor Intervention Trial," *JAMA* 257 (1987):943–47. See table 1.

26. R. R. Butrum et al., "NCI Dietary Guidelines Rationale," *American Journal of Clinical Nutrition* 48 (1988):888–95

27. Durk Pearson and Sandy Shaw, *Life Extension: A Practical Scientific Approach* (New York: Warner Books, 1983); Weil, *Spontaneous Healing*, pp. 159–60.

28. "We're Still Taking Our Beta-Carotene," *Wellness Letter,* (University of California at Berkeley) vol. 10, no. 10 (July 1994).

29. Rebecca Voelker, "Recommendations for Antioxidants: How Much Evidence Is Enough?" *JAMA* 271 (1994):1148–49.

30. "We're Still Taking Our Beta-Carotene."

31. Coronary Drug Project Research Group, "The Coronary Drug Project: Findings Learning to Further Modifications of Its Protocol with Respect to Dextrothyroxine," *JAMA* 220 (1972):996–1008.

32. Thomas J. Moore, *Deadly Medicine* (New York: Simon & Schuster, 1995), pp. 208–32.

5. DRUGS AND BEHAVIOR

1. Stephen Fried, "Prescription for Disaster," *Washington Post Magazine*, April 3, 1994, p. 13.

2. *Physicians' Desk Reference.*

3. S. J. Lensgraf and A. R. Favazza, "Antidepressent-Induced Mania," *American Journal of Psychiatry* 147 (1990):1569.

4. *Physicians' Desk Reference.*

5. "Prozac 6% Scripts Growth Pleasing but Not Satisfactory, Lilly Says," FDC Reports, *The Pink Sheet,* May 27, 1996.

6. *Grundberg v. The Upjohn Co.* (C.D.Utah, 1991) 137 F.R.D. 372.

7. *State of Missouri v. Lila Wacaser,* Circuit Court of Platt County,

Missouri, CR187-1073FX, transcript of videotaped deposition of William S. Barry, p.52.

8. Goodman and Gilman, pp. 431ff.

9. E. Christopher Iliades, "Doctor and Addict," *Washington Post*, September 3, 1996, Health section; and personal interview.

10. U.S. Department of Health and Human Services, "Preliminary Estimates from the Drug Abuse Warning Network," Advanced Report no. 11, November 1995, p. 50.

11. U.S. Department of Health and Human Services, *National Household Survey on Drug Abuse: Population Estimates 1994* (Rockville, Md.: Public Health Service, 1995).

12. M. Clark et al., "The Prisoners of Pills," *Newsweek*, April 24, 1978, p. 11.

13. "Kitty Dukakis Dependent on Amphetamines for 26 Years," *New York Times,* July 9, 1987.

14. Colleen O'Connor, "Bad Medical Advice for Rehnquist?" *Newsweek,* August 25, 1986, p. 32.

15. D. A. Ciraulo, "Abuse Potential of Benzodiazepines," *Bulletin of the New York Academy of Sciences* 61 (1985):728-41.

16. B. Dickinson et al., "Alprazolam Use and Dependence: A Retrospective Analysis of 30 Cases of Withdrawal," *Western Journal of Medicine* 152 (1990):604–8.

17. Goodman and Gilman, p. 374.

18. American Psychiatric Association, *Diagnostic and Statistical Manual of Mental Disorders* (DSM-IV), 4th ed., (Washington, D.C.: American Psychiatric Association, 1994), p. 181.

19. Ibid., pp. 182–83.

20. D. F. Musto, "Iatrogenic Addiction: The Problem, Its Definition and History," *Bulletin of the New York Academy of Medicine* 61 (1985):694–705.

21. Peter R. Breggin, *Talking Back to Prozac* (New York: St. Martin's Press, 1994).

22. Carl Salzman, *Benzodiazepine Dependence, Toxicity and Abuse: A Task Force Report of the American Psychiatric Association* (Washington, D.C.: American Psychiatric Association, 1990).

23. B. M. Maletzky, "Addiction to Propoxyphene (Darvon): A Second Look," *International Journal of the Addictions* 9 (1974):775–84; S. B. Soumerai, "Effect of Government and Commercial Warnings on Reducing Prescription Misuse: The Case of Propoxyphene," *American Journal of Public Health* 77 (1987:) 1518–23.

24. C. G. Moertel et al., "A Comparative Evaluation of Marketed Analgesic Drugs," *New England Journal of Medicine* 286 (1972):813.

25. "Tramadol for Pain," *Medical Sciences Bulletin*, April 1995.

26. U.S. Department of Health and Human Services, Food and Drug Administration, "New Labeling for Rx Pain Reliever, Tramadol," press release, April 3, 1996.

6. THE THREAT TO CELLS

1. Insight Team of the Sunday *Times* of London, *Suffer the Children: The Story of Thalidomide* (New York: Viking Press, 1979), details from chaps. 1, 6, and 7.

2. Morton Mintz, *By Prescription Only* (Boston: Beacon Press, 1967), p. 261.

3. *Physicians' Desk Reference*. These are "Pregnancy Category A" drugs.

4. Author's computer scan of the *Physicians' Desk Reference*, CD-ROM version.

5. A. Giroud et al., "Thalidomide and Congenital Abnormalities," *Lancet* 2 (1962):298.

6. *Physicians' Desk Reference*.

7. Calculated by the author from a computer search of the *Physicians' Desk Reference*. A "drug" is any chemical agent listed in this volume. An oral and IV drug would be listed twice. A similar or identical drug with a different manufacturer would also be listed twice. For example, five of six drugs safe in human studies are very similiar thyroid hormone replacements.

8. B. A. Miller et al., *SEER Cancer Statistics Review: 1973–1990,*

National Cancer Institute, NIH Publ. no. 93-2789, 1993. For 1993, it was 1.1 million new cases and 526,000 estimated deaths.

9. Smoking also gets blamed in another 20 to 25 percent of cases among former smokers when no current damage is clinically evident.

10. C. D. Klaassen et al., eds., *Casarett & Doull's Toxicology: The Basic Science of Poisons* (New York: McGraw-Hill), 1996, p. 226.

11. A. H. Wylie, "Apoptosis: Cell Death in Tissue Regulation," *Journal of Pathology* 153 (1987):313–16.

12. Robert Doll and Richard Peto, "Avoidable Risks of Cancer in the United States," *Journal of the National Cancer Institute* 6 (1981):1194–1268. Because drugs and radiation are given simultaneously in cancer treatment, it is difficult to separate the two factors. Doll and Peto guess that radiation might account for half of the deaths.

13. T. S. Davies and A. Monro, "Marketed Human Pharmaceuticals Reported to Be Tumorigenic in Rodents," *Journal of the American College of Toxicology* 14 (1995):90–107.

14. Ibid., appendix.

15. For this estimate, we must rely on the assumption that the drugs too old to have undergone modern systematic testing carry about the same risk as those for which results are available.

16. Klaassen et al., *Casarett & Doull's Toxicology,* p. 31 in the 4th ed. In the 5th ed., another exception was added—benzene, a curious choice since it is implicated in other animal toxicology summaries, such as L. S. Gold, "Extrapolation of Carcinogenicity Between Species: Qualitative and Quantitative Factors," *Risk Analysis* 12 (1992):579–88.

17. Gold, "Extrapolation of Carcinogenicity."

18. In every known human cancer where benign growths are observed, malignant tumors also occur.

19. Klaassen et al., *Casarett & Doull's Toxicology,* 244.

20. Ibid., pp. 672–73. While it is reasonably clear dioxin does not have in humans the enormously toxic properties seen in animals,

questions remain about whether it can cause birth defects or has mutagenic effects.

21. L. S. Gold, "The Importance of Data on Mechanism of Carcinogenesis in Efforts to Predict Low-Dose Human Risks," *Risk Analysis* 13 (1993):399–401.

22. In toxicology testing, the conversion from animal to human exposure is achieved by comparing the surface area of the two species. An earlier standard used just body weight but has been largely abandoned because it makes chemicals appear to be about ten times safer.

23. *Physicians' Desk Reference*.

24. Ibid. The carcinogenic effects were reported at about twice the maximum human dose by the body weight standard, but at less than the human dose using the more conservative standard of surface area.

25. Ibid.

26. Ibid.

27. Klaassen et al., *Casarett & Doull's Toxicology*, 4th ed., p. 38.

28. Ibid.

29. U. S. Department of Health and Human Services, *Seventh Annual Report on Carcinogens: Summary 1995* (Rockville, Md.: Technical Resources, 1994).

30. A. L. Herbst et al., "Adenocarcinoma of the Vagina," *New England Journal of Medicine* 284 (1971):878–81.

31. D. B. Dutton, *Worse Than the Disease: Pitfalls of Medical Progress* (New York: Cambridge University Press, 1988), chap. 3.

32. A. D. Langmuir, "New Environmental Factor in Congenital Disease," *New England Journal of Medicine* 284 (1971): 912–13.

33. Dutton, *Worse Than the Disease*, p. 74. Four years later, one pediatrician told a U.S. Senate hearing that he couldn't persuade colleagues who were obstetricians to stop prescribing DES (p. 74).

34. D. H. Mills, "Prenatal Diethylstilbestrol and Vaginal Cancer in Offspring," *JAMA* 229 (1974):472–73.

35. A. L. Herbst, "The Epidemiology of Vaginal and Clear Cell Adenocarcinoma," in A. L. Herbst, and Howard Bern, eds., *Developmental Effects of DES in Pregnancy* (New York: Thieme-Stratton, 1981).

36. S. J. Robboy et al., "Pathologic Findings in Young Women Enrolled in the National Cooperative Diethylstilbestrol Adenosis (DESAD) Project," *Obstetrics & Gynecology* 53 (1979): 309–17; W. B. Gill et at., "Male Genital Tract Changes in Humans Following Intrauterine Exposure to Diethylstilbestrol," in Herbst and Bern, *Developmental Effects*, p. 103.

37. N. S. Weiss et al., "Increasing Incidence of Endometrial Cancer in the United States," *New England Journal of Medicine* 294 (1976):1259–62; D. C. Smith et al., "Association of Exogenous Estrogen and Endometrial Carcinoma," *New England Journal of Medicine* 293 (1975):1164–67; H. K. Ziel and W. D. Finkle, "Increased Risk of Endometrial Carcinoma Among Users of Conjugated Estrogens," *New England Journal of Medicine* 293 (1975):1167–70.

38. T. M. Mack et al., "Estrogens and Endometrial Cancer in a Retirement Community," *New England Journal of Medicine* 294 (1976):1262–67; T. W. McDonald et al., "Exogenous Estrogen and Endometrial Carcinoma: Case-Control and Incidence Study," *American Journal of Obstetrics and Gynecology* 127 (1976):572–80.

39. Hershel Jick et al., "The Epidemic of Endometrial Cancer: A Commentary," *American Journal of Public Health* 70 (1980):264–67.

40. N. S. Weiss, personal communication.

41. G. S. Omenn et al., "Effects of a Combination of Beta Carotene and Vitamin A on Lung Cancer and Cardiovascular Disease," *New England Journal of Medicine* 334 (1996):1150–55. From table 2, the placebo group rate for asbestos workers, 97 percent of whom had a history of cigarette smoking.

42. B. A. Miller et al., *SEER Cancer Statistics Review: 1973–1990*. (Bethesda, MD.: National Cancer Institute, 1993).

43. E. Heimiki et al., "Prescribing of Noncontraceptive Estrogens and Progestins in the United States, 1974–1986," *American Journal of Public Health* 78 (1988):1479–81.

44. I. Persson et al., "Risk of Endometrial Cancer After Treatment with Oestrogens Alone or in Conjunction with Progestogens: Results of a Prospective Study," *BMJ* 298 (1989):147–151; L. F. Voigt et al., "Progestogen Supplementation of Exogenous Oestrogens and the Risk of Endometrial Cancer," *Lancet* 338 (1991):274–77.

45. *Physicians' Desk Reference.*

46. B. E. Henderson et al., "Estrogens as a Cause of Human Cancer: The Richard and Hinda Rosenthal Foundation Award Lecture," *Cancer Research* 48 (1988):246–53. Because breast cancer is so much more common than endometrial cancer, it is harder to achieve conclusive findings, even if the danger is greater.

47. American College of Physicians, "Guidelines for Counseling Postmenopausal Women About Preventive Hormone Therapy," *Annals of Internal Medicine* 117 (1992):1038–41; D. Grady et al., "Hormone Therapy to Prevent Disease and Prolong Life in Postmenopausal Women," *Annals of Internal Medicine* 117 (1992):1016–37.

48. Klaassen et al., *Casarett & Doull's Toxicology*, 5th ed., p. 29.

49. P. Greenwald and E. J. Sondik, *Cancer Control: Objectives for the Nation: 1985-2000,* NCI Monographs, no. 2, 1986. A team of experts used a computer model to project a 50 percent drop in the cancer death rate by the year 2000. They thought achieving these goals required only a broader application of known treatments and a modest reduction in cigarette smoking.

50. Goodman and Gilman, p. 1134. Because of reporting problems discussed elsewhere, I suspect the real incidence was higher.

51. *Physicians' Desk Reference.*

52. F. W. Madison and T. L. Squier, "The Etiology of Primary Granulocytopenia," *JAMA* 102 (1934):755–59.

53. L. K. Hine et al., "Mortality Resulting from Blood Dyscrasias

in the United States, 1984," *American Journal of Medicine* 8 (1990):151–53.

54. *Physicians' Desk Reference.*

55. Ibid.

56. Ibid.

7. THE SYSTEM

1. Office of the President of the United States, *Budget of the United States Government, Fiscal Year 1991* (Washington, D.C.: Government Printing Office, 1990), p. A-603. See Personnel Summary, total of compensable work years. Letter to the author from Vincent Guinee, M.D., of the Division of Pharmacovigilance and Epidemiology, Food and Drug Administration, U.S. Department of Health and Human Services, May 19, 1997.

2. Joseph DiMasi, "Success Rates for New Drugs Entering Clinical Testing in the United States," *Clinical Pharmacology & Therapeutics* 58 (1995):1–14.

3. O. M. Bakke et al., "Drug Discontinuations in the United Kingdom and the United States, 1964 to 1983: Issues of Safety," *Clinical Pharmacology & Therapeutics* 35 (1984):559–67. However, note that the newer drugs, subject to more extensive initial testing, were only on the market an average of four years before withdrawal.

4. Joseph A. DiMasi et al., "R & D Costs, Innovative Output, and Firm Size in the Pharmaceutical Industry," *International Journal of the Economics of Business* 2 (1995):201–19.

5. M. F. Shapiro, "Scientific Misconduct in Investigational Drug Trials," *New England Journal of Medicine* 312 (1985):731–36. It is not comforting that this survey found 11.5 percent of trials had serious deficiencies.

6. U.S. General Accounting Office, *FDA Drug Approval: Review Time Has Decreased in Recent Years,* GAO/PEMD-96-1 (Washington, D.C.: General Accounting Office, 1996). In this report, the sixteen-month approval time was achieved only for

drugs with major therapeutic benefit in 1992. By 1996, most drugs were meeting this standard. David A. Kessler et al., "Approval of New Drugs in the United States: Comparison with the United Kingdom, Germany, and Japan," *JAMA* 276 (1996):1826–31.

7. Thomas J. Moore, *Deadly Medicine* (New York: Simon & Schuster, 1995), p. 110.

8. U.S. Department of Health and Human Services, Food and Drug Administration, "New Labeling for Rx Pain Reliever Tramdol," Talk Paper (press release), April 3, 1996.

9. *Physicians' Desk Reference.*

10. U.S. Department of Health and Human Services, Food and Drug Administration, Advisory Committee on Endocrine and Metabolic Drugs, February 19, 1987.

11. U.S. General Accounting Office, *FDA Drug Review: Postapproval Risks 1976–85,* GAO/PEMD-90-15 (Washington, D.C.: General Accounting Office, 1990).

12. Some of these employees may spend about 5 percent of their time monitoring the safety of approved drugs, according to unpublished FDA budget studies obtained by the author. They also must review about fifty simpler applications for new medical uses of already approved drugs.

13. Unpublished budget summaries for Fiscal Year 1995 provided by the Food and Drug Administration.

14. D. E. Knapp et al.,. *Annual Adverse Drug Experience Report: 1995,* Surveillance and Data Processing Branch, Division of Pharmacovigilance and Epidemiology, Center for Drug Evaluation and Research, Food and Drug Administration, n.d.

15. Kevin L. Ropp, "MedWatch: On the Lookout for Medical Product Problems," *FDA Consumer* Special Report, 2nd ed., *From Test Tube to Patient: New Drug Development in the United States,* January 1995, p. 43.

16. U.S. Department of Health and Human Services, Food and Drug Administration, "Manoplax," press release, April 26, 1993.

17. D. S. Echt et al., "Mortality and Morbidity in Patients Re-

ceiving Encainide, Flecainide, or Placebo," *New England Journal of Medicine* 324 (1991):781–88.

18. *Physicians' Desk Reference.*

19. John Lechus, Office of Regulatory Affairs, Food and Drug Administration, interview. FDA field inspectors often inspect other kinds of facilities—such as food-processing plants. The 73 figure is full-time-equivalent employees. Including support, management, and other workers, the total is the equivalent of 131. Another 144 full-time-equivalent employees obtain drugs on the open market and analyze their content.

20. U.S. Department of Health and Human Services, Food and Drug Administration, "Lilly Reaches Compliance Agreement with FDA," Talk Paper (press release), November 3, 1989.

21. Warner-Lambert Co., annual reports.

22. *The Pink Sheet,* FDC Reports, October 9, 1995, p. 15.

23. S. M. Wilcox, et al., "Inappropriate Drug Prescribing in the Community-Dwelling Elderly," *JAMA* 272 (1992):292–96.

24. J. H. Gurwitz, "Suboptimal Medication Use in the Elderly: The Tip of the Iceberg," *JAMA* 272 (1994):316–17.

25. A. E. Stuck et al., "Inappropriate Medication Use in Community-Residing Older Persons," *Archives of Internal Medicine* 154 (1994):2195–200.

26. U.S. General Accounting Office, *Many Still Receive Potentially Harmful Drugs Despite Recent Improvements.* GAO/HEHS-95-152 (Washington, D.C.: General Accounting Office, 1995).

27. N. J. Cavuto et al., "Pharmacies and Prevention of Potentially Fatal Drug Interactions," *JAMA* 275 (1996):1086.

28. J. A. Cramer et al., "How Often is Medication Taken as Prescribed?" *JAMA* 261 (1989):3273–77.

29. Adnan Dajani, "Adherence to Physicians' Instructions as a Factor in Managing Streptococcal Pharyngitis," *Pediatrics,* June 1996, suppl. 2, pp. 976–80.

30. C. S. Rand and R. A. Wise, "Measuring Adherence to Asthma Medication Regimens," *American Journal of Respiratory and Critical Care Medicine* (1994) 249(2 Pt 2):S69–76.

8. PAIN

1. United States Senate, Committee on Labor and Human Resources, *Hearing on S. 1477,* February 21, 1996, p. 6.

2. James F. Fries, "NSAID Gastropathy: The Second Most Deadly Rheumatic Disease?" *Journal of Rheumatology* 18 (1991), suppl. 28, pp. 6–10. This is a conservative estimate that omits all the middle-ages athletes without arthritis taking anti-inflammatory drugs. There are published estimates of 200,000 cases a year.

3. Ivan T. Borda and Raymond S. Koff, *NSAIDS: A Profile of Adverse Effects* (Philadelphia: Hanley & Belfus, 1992), p.1. The adverse reactions reported were not only the largest in total number; they were more than expected from the volume of prescriptions.

4. D. E. Knapp et al., *Annual Adverse Drug Experience Report: 1995,* Surveillance and Data Processing Branch, Division of Pharmacovigilance and Epidemiology, Food and Drug Administration, n.d.

5. Borda and Koff, *NSAIDS,* p. xi.

6. Sidney M. Wolfe, "Differences in the Number of Drug Safety Withdrawals: United States, United Kingdom, Germany, France, 1970–1992." Washington, D.C.: Public Citizen Health Research Group, February 2, 1995. Additional studies and details are cited later.

7. Fries, *NSAID Gastropathy.*

8. Ibid.

9. Goodman and Gilman, chap. 27. There is little debate whether anti-inflammatory drugs inhibit the synthesis of prostaglandins; however, some researchers question whether this is the most important mechanism by which the drugs achieve their anti-inflammatory effect.

10. Steroid hormones such as cortisone also suppress the inflammation response throughout the body. These aspirinlike anti-inflammatory drugs are called "nonsteroidal" anti-inflammatory drugs, or, abbreviated, NSAID.

11. W. G. Clark et al., *Goth's Medical Pharmacology* (St. Louis: Mosby Year Book, 1992), p. 226.

12. S. H. Roth, "Non-Steroidal Anti-Inflammatory Drug Gastropathy: Recognition and Response," *Archives of Internal Medicine* 147 (1987):2093–100

13. G. R. Silvoso et al., "Incidence of Gastric Lesions in Patients with Rheumatic Disease on Chronic Aspirin Therapy," *Annals of Internal Medicine* 91 (1979):517–20.

14. G. Singh et al., "Comparative Toxicity of Non-Steroidal Anti-Inflammatory Agents," *Pharmaceutical Therapeutics* 62 (1994):175–91.

15. G. S. Gies et al., "Prevalence of Mucosal Lesions in the Stomach and Duodenum Due to Chronic Use of NSAID in Patients with Rheumatoid Arthritis or Osteoarthritis," *Journal of Rheumatology* 18 (1991), suppl. 28, pp. 11–14.

16. J. A. Melogomes et al., "Double-Blind Comparison of Efficacy and Gastroduodenal Safety of Diclofenac/Misoprostol, Proxicam, and Naproxen in the Treatment of Osteoarthritis," *Annals of Rheumatic Disease* 52 (1993):881–85.

17. B. S. Bloom, "Direct Medical Costs of Disease and Gastrointestinal Side Effects During Treatment for Arthritis," *American Journal of Medicine* 84 (1988), suppl. 2A, pp. 20–24.

18. This figure is from the FDA-approved class warning that appears on the disclosure label of drugs in this class such as ibuprofen, ketoprofen, naproxen, and priroxicam.

19. C. P. Armstrong and A. L. Blower. "Non-Steroidal Anti-Inflammatory Drugs and Life-Threatening Complications of Peptic Ulceration," *Gut* 28 (1987):727–32.

20. Bloom, "Direct Medical Costs."

21. Walter E. Smalley, "Excess Costs from Gastrointestinal Disease Associated with Non-Steroidal Anti-Inflammatory Drugs," *Journal of General Internal Medicine* 11 (1996):461–69.

22. J. C. Krance, *Historical Medical Classics Involving New Drugs* (Baltimore: Williams & Wilkins Co., 1974), p. 41.

23. O. M. Bakke et al., "Drug Safety Discontinuations in the United Kingdom, the United States, and Spain from 1974 through 1993," *Clinical Pharmacology & Therapeutics* 58

(1995):108–17; O. M. Bakke et al., "Drug Discontinuations in the United Kingdom and the United States, 1964 to 1983: Issues of Safety," *Clinical Pharmacology & Therapeutics* 35 (1984):559–67; Sidney M. Wolfe, "Differences in the Number of Drug Safety Withdrawals," Public Citizen Health Research Group, February 2, 1995.

24. John Abraham, *Science, Politics, and the Pharmaceutical Industry* (New York: St. Martin's Press, 1995), p. 138.

25. In the case of a drug that both relieves symptoms and causes symptoms, that is the essence of the patient decision to discontinue. The discontinuation rate is for Prozac, Paxil, and Zoloft.

26. Abraham, *Science, Politics, and the Pharmaceutical Industry*, p. 138.

27. James F. Fries, "Postmarketing Drug Surveillance: Are Our Priorities Right?" *Journal of Rheumatology* 15 (1988):389–90.

28. *Physicians' Desk Reference.*

29. G. Singh et al., "Gastrointestinal Tract Complications of Non-steroidal Anti-inflammatory Drug Treatment in Rheumatoid Arthritis," *Archives of Internal Medicine* 156 (1996):1530–36.

30. This is the recommendation of the October 23, 1995, guidelines from the American College of Rheumatology.

31. A. C. Jones et al., "Non-Steroidal Anti-Inflammatory Drug Usage and Requirement in Elderly Acute Hospital Admissions," *British Journal of Rheumatology* 31 (1992):45–48.

32. S. H. Roth, "NSAIDs: Risk-Benefit Versus Cost-Benefit," *Drug Information Journal* 22 (1988):477–81.

33. "UK Medical Chief Calls for Risk Debate," *Scrip*, October 4, 1996.

34. CVS Pharmacy, printed instructions for Oruvail, obtained on November 7, 1996.

35. All these warnings are from the listed drugs in the 1996 *Physicians' Desk Reference.*

9. SLEEP

1. Harold H. Morris, "You Don't Have to Be a Neuroscientist to

Forget Everything with Triazolam—But It Helps." Letter in response to reader comments. *JAMA* 259 (1988):351–52.

2. Harold H. Morris and Melinda L. Estes, "Traveler's Amnesia: Transient Global Amnesia Secondary to Triazolam," *JAMA* 258 (1987):945–46.

3. Kim Cobb, "The Sleep Merchants: The Halcion Story," *Houston Chronicle,* September 11–14, 1994.

4. *Upjohn v. Freeman* (Tex. App., 1994) 885 S.W.2d 538. In this tangled legal case, a jury found Upjohn grossly negligent and awarded Freeman's family $1.8 million, but the appellate court reversed the verdict on technical legal grounds.

5. William S. Barry. Videotaped deposition played February 1, 1992, in *State of Missouri v. Nila Wacaser,* Case Number CR187-1073FX, Circuit Court of Platt County, p. 52.

6. As listed in Physicians' Desk Reference, which omits many generic drugs. However, the same chemical molecule sold in different forms—such as short-acting and sustained release—was counted as two separate drugs, as were various forms and combinations of aspirin.

7. Goodman and Gilman, p. 453.

8. Ibid.; W. G. Clark et al., *Goth's Medical Pharmacology* (St. Louis: Mosby Year Book, 1992), pp. 266–67.

9. Ibid., Fig. 29-1, p. 270.

10. Ibid.

11. Committee on the Safety of Medicines, paper presented to the other European Community on Proprietary Medicinal Products, 1991.

12. Committee on the Safety of Medicines, "A Re-Evaluation of the Safety of Triazolam," December 1991, unpublished.

13. Upjohn CEO Theodore Cooper declared in 1991 that the discrepancy was a "transcription error." However, an FDA investigation of Protocol 321 declared that this explanation was "false and misleading." However, the principal investigator, Harold Oster, apparently never even saw the final results.

14. Steven R. Reed, "Halcion Research Called Into Question,"

Houston Chronicle, September 12, 1994. U.S. Department of Health and Human Services, Food and Drug Administration, Office of Health Affairs, "Disqualified/Restricted/Assurances List for Clinical Investigators, as of August 22, 1997."

15. Department of Health and Human Services, Food and Drug Administration, "The Establishment Inspection Report Dated December 1991 and March 3–4, 1992, for Upjohn Company, Kalamazoo, MI," p. 9.

16. Cees van der Kroef, "Reactions to Triazolam," *Lancet* 2 (1979):526.

17. F. J. Ayd et al., "Behavioural Reactions to Triazolam," *Lancet* 2 (1979):1018.

18. FDA report, p. 5.

19. British Broadcasting Corporation, *Panorama,* October 14, 1991.

20. FDA report, p. 5.

21. John Abraham and Julie Sheppard, "Conflicting Scientific Expertise in British and American Medicines Control." Report to the ESRC Ref R000221470, June 1996, p. 7.

22. Ibid., p. 8.

23. Clark, *Goth's Medical Pharmacology,* Fig. 29-1, p. 270.

24. FDA report, p. 3.

25. *Physicians' Desk Reference,* 1984 ed., p. 2027. The original package insert said, "It is recommended that Halcion not be prescribed in quantities exceeding a one-month supply."

26. At the time Leber took this action, it was called the Division of Epidemiology and Biostatistics.

27. Diane K. Wysowski and David Barash, "Adverse Behavioral Reactions Attributed to Triazolam in the Food and Drug Administration's Spontaneous Reporting System," *Archives of Internal Medicine* 151 (1991):2003–8.

28. FDA report, p. 33.

29. Ibid., p. 6.

30. Ibid.

31. Ibid., p. 52.

32. Technically, it is the doctor who has been warned and, as a learned intermediary, is responsible for passing this information on to the consumer.

33. However, the *International Herald Tribune* (Paris) had published the same story. Upjohn also sued the BBC for the *Panorama* program.

34. FDA report, p. 8.

35. U.S. Department of Health and Human Services, Food and Drug Administration, "Report of the Halcion Task Force," May 29, 1996, p. ii.

36. The Upjohn Co., "Upjohn Wins Libel Trial in U.K.," PR newswire, May 27, 1994.

37. Raymond A. Bauer and Lawrence Wortzel, "Doctor's Choice: The Physician and His Source of Information About Drugs," *Journal of Marketing Research III* (1966):40–47. Jerry Avorn et al., "Scientific versus Commercial Sources of Influence on the Prescribing Behavior of Physicians," *American Journal of Medicine* 73 (1982):4–8.

38. Thomas Maeder, *Adverse Reactions* (New York: William Morrow & Co., 1994).

39. John A. Byrne, *Informed Consent* (New York: McGraw-Hill, 1996).

40. Morton Mintz, *At Any Cost* (New York: Pantheon Books, 1985).

41. Thomas J. Moore, *Deadly Medicine* (New York: Simon & Schuster,1995).

10. THE DOCTOR'S OFFICE.

1. S. M. Schappert, "National Ambulatory Medical Care Survey: 1990 Summary," *Advance Data from Vital and Health Statistics of the National Center for Health Statistics,* no. 213, April 30, 1992; National Center for Health Statistics.

2. The Keystone Center, *Action Plan for the Provision of Useful Prescription Medicine Information* (Keystone, Colo.: Keystone Center, 1996), p. 6. C. R. Nekson, "Drug Utilization in Office

Practice: National Ambulatory Medical Care Survey, 1990," *Advance Data from Vital and Health Statistics of the Centers for Disease Control and Prevention,* no. 232, March 25, 1993, National Center for Health Statistics.

3. Schappert, "National Ambulatory Medical Care Survey."

4. J. N. Katz et al., "Informed Consent and the Prescription of Nonsteroidal Anti-inflammatory Drugs," *Arthritis and Rheumatism* 35 (1992):1257–63.

5. L. A. Morris et al., "Counseling Patients About Prescribed Medication: 12-Year Trends," *Medical Care* (1997) (in press).

6. President's Commission for the Study of Ethical Problems in Medicine and Biomedical and Behavioral Research, *Making Health Care Decisions* (Washington, D.C.: Government Printing Office, 1982).

7. Ibid., p. 54.

8. R. S. Litman et al., "Parental Knowledge and Attitudes Toward Discussing the Risk of Death from Anesthesia," *Pediatric Anesthesia* 77 (1993):256–60.

9. R. R. Faden et al., "Disclosure of Information to Patients in Medical Care," *Medical Care* 19 (1981):718–33.

10. Goodman and Gilman, p. 407.

11. Ibid.

12. American Psychiatric Association, *Tardive Dyskinesia,* APA Task Force Report no. 18. (Washington, D.C.: American Psychiatric Association, 1979).

13. P. R. Benson, "Informed Consent: Drug Information Disclosed to Patients Prescribed Antipsychotic Medication," *Journal of Nervous and Mental Disease* 172 (1984):642–53.

14. M. R. Munetz, "Overcoming Resistance to Talking to Patients About Tardive Dyskinesia," *Hospital and Community Psychiatry* 36 (1985):283–87.

15. President's Commission, *Making Health Care Decisions,* p. 46.

16. Ibid. See the beginning of the chapter "Drugs and Behavior."

17. W. E. Sanders, letters to the editor, *Washington Post Magazine,* May 22, 1994.

18. Peter R. Breggin, *Toxic Psychiatry* (New York: St. Martin's Press, 1992), p. 77.

19. Ibid. See chaps. 7 and 19.

20. U.S. Department of Health and Human Services, Food and Drug Administration, "Prescription Drug Products: Patient Package Inserts," *Federal Register,* September 12, 1980, p. 60748.

21. U.S. Department of Health and Human Services, Food and Drug Administration, "FDA Announces Patient Education Program," statement, August 23, 1995.

22. "Minority Report of the AMA, AAFP, and ACOG to the Action Plan for Provision of Useful Prescription Medicine Information," December 12, 1996, unpublished.

23. Ibid.

24. Alan F. Holmer, Pharmaceutical Research and Manufacturers of America, letter of December 10, 1996, in response to a preliminary report on voluntary program of prescription information.

25. "Minority Report of the AMA."

26. *Physicians' Desk Reference.*

27. Ibid.

28. Goodman and Gilman, pp. 1348–50.

29. W. A. Ray et al., "Benzodiazepines of Long and Short Elimination Half-Life and the Risk of Hip Fracture," *JAMA* 262 (1989):3303–7.

30. *Hattie Rotan v. Seymour Greenbaum,* 273 F.2d 830; 107 U.S. App. D.C.16.

31. R. Y. Lin, "A Perspective on Penicillin Allergy," *Archives of Internal Medicine* 152 (1992):930–37.

32. Ibid.

33. A. G. Mainous, "Antibiotics and Upper Respiratory Infection: Do Some Folks Think There Is a Cure for the Common Cold?" *Journal of Family Practice* 42 (1996):357–61.

34. S. B. Soumerai and H. L. Lipton, "Evaluating and Improving Physician Prescribing Practices," in B. L. Strom, *Pharmacoepidemiology* (New York: John Wiley & Sons, 1994), p. 396.

35. Mainous, "Antibiotics and Upper Respiratory Infection."

36. J. M. Piper, "Maternal Use of Prescribed Drugs Associated with Recognized Fetal Adverse Drug Reactions," *American Journal of Obstetrics and Gynecology* 159 (1988):1173–77

37. W. A. Ray et al., "Prescribing of Tetracycline to Children Less than 8 Years Old," *JAMA* 237 (1977):2069–74.

38. W. S. Aronow, "Prevalence of Appropriate and Inappropriate Indications for Use of Digoxin in Older Patients at the Time of Admission to a Nursing Home," *Journal of the American Geriatric Society*, 44 (1996):588–90.

39. R. H. Grimm et al., "Evaluation and Patient-Care Protocol Use by Various Providers," *New England Journal of Medicine* 292 (1975):507–11.

40. G. O. Barnet et al., "Quality Assurance Through Automated Monitoring and Current Feedback Using a Computer-Based Medical Information System," *Medical Care* 21 (1978):500–509. With computerized reminders, the rate of patients not contacted declined to 3 percent, and then rose back to 10 percent again at the end of the program.

41. Cardiac Arrhythmia Suppression Trial (CAST) Investigators, "Preliminary Report: Effect of Encainide and Flecainide on Mortality in a Randomized Clinical Trial After Myocardial Infarction," *New England Journal of Medicine* 321 (1989):406–12.

42. James A. Reiffel et al., "Physician Attitudes Towards the Use of Type IC Antiarrhythmics After the Cardiac Arrhythmia Suppression Trial (CAST)," *American Journal of Cardiology* 66 (1990):1262–64.

43. S. B. Soumerai, "Adverse Outcomes of Underuse of Beta-Blockers in Elderly Survivors of Acute Myocardial Infarction," *JAMA* 277 (1997):115–21.

44. Ibid.

45. M. Olfson and H. A. Pincus, "Use of Benzodiazepines in the Community," *Archives of Internal Medicine* 154 (1994):1235–40.

46. Ibid.

47. Seven years after the warning was issued, the FDA proposed

in 1997 that Seldane be withdrawn from the market because the same company had just marketed a safer alternative. However, it took no action against Hismanal, which has the same risks as Seldane, and ignored the fact that Claritin, a safer alternative, had been available for several years.

48. *Physicians' Desk Reference.*

49. A truly alert doctor might wonder whether the differences between the two groups could have occurred as a result of chance. The FDA and 3M introduced this further confusion by incorrectly separating the results for Tambocor from the overall results for two drugs, Tambocor and Enkaid. In the trial, the valid findings were for both drugs combined.

50. Thomas Maeder, *Adverse Reactions* (New York: William Morrow & Co., 1994), P. 189.

51. D. Ross-Degnan et al., "Examining Product Risk in Context: Market Withdrawal of Zomepirac Sodium as a Case Study," *JAMA* 270 (1993):1937–42.

52. Soumerai and Lipton, "Evaluating and Improving Physician Prescribing Practices," p. 402.

11. FIXING THE SYSTEM

1. U.S. Congress, Office of Technology Assessment, *Pharmaceutical R & D: Costs, Risks and Rewards* (Washington, D.C.: Government Printing Office, 1993).

2. John Schwartz, "FDA Often Blamed for Problems that Aren't the Agency's Fault," *Washington Post,* July 15, 1996.

3. P. F. Reinstein and J. I. Robinson, "Annual Adverse Drug Experience Report, 1994," Surveillance Section, Division of Pharmacovigilance and Epidemiology, Food and Drug Administration, n.d.

4. This is the leading or most common approved medical use. Prozac, for example, is also approved for treating obsessive-compulsive disorder.

5. Reinstein and Robinson, "Annual Adverse Drug Experience Report."

6. J. L. Warren et al., "Hospitalizations with Adverse Events

Caused by Digitalis Therapy Among Elderly Medicare Beneficiaries," *Archives of Internal Medicine* 154 (1994):1482–87.

7. Ibid.

8. The total staff of the Division of Pharmacovigilance and Epidemiology was fifty-four persons in 1997. The other employees were involved in data processing for the reports, and in interviewing and evaluating individual reports for consistency and possible trends.

9. Thomas J. Moore, *Research Policy Brief: Monitoring and Safety of Drugs in the Marketplace* (Washington, D.C.: Center for Health Policy Research, 1997).

10. J. A. DiMasi, "Success Rates for New Drugs Entering Clinical Testing in the United States," *Clinical Pharmacology & Therapeutics* 58 (1995):1–14.

11. *Physicians' Desk Reference.*

12. American Psychiatric Association, *Tardive Dyskinesia,* APA Task Force Report no. 18 (Washington, D.C.: American Psychiatric Association, 1979).

13. *Physicians' Desk Reference;* R. K. Shrivastava et al., "Long-Term Safety and Clinical Acceptability of Venlafaxine and Imipramine in Outpatients with Major Depression," *Journal of Clinical Psychopharmacology* 14 (1994):322–29. Here is an example of an uncontrolled long-term safety study that shows very little since only 34 percent of the patients were still taking the drug after one year. Such uncontrolled studies exist for other antidepressants.

14. J. Shepard et al., "Prevention of Coronary Heart Disease with Pravastatin in Men with Hypercholesterolemia," *New England Journal of Medicine* 333 (1995):1301–7; F. M. Sacks et al., "The Effect of Pravastatin or Coronary Events After Myocardial Infarction in Patients with Average Cholesterol Levels," *New England Journal of Medicine* 335 (1996):1001–9.

15. M. F. Oliver, "W.H.O. Cooperative Trial on Primary Prevention of Ischaemic Heart Disease Using Clofibrate to Lower Serum Cholesterol: Mortality Follow-Up," *Lancet* 2 (1980):379–85.

16. The drug is still on the market with a warning in the product disclosure label that it increased the death rate.

17. University Group Diabetes Program Investigators, "University Group Diabetes Program," *Diabetes* 19 (1970), suppl. 2, pt. 1 (Design), pt. 2 (Mortality Results).

18. American Diabetes Association, statement released October 27, 1970.

19. American Diabetes Association, "New Recommendations to Lower the Diabetes Diagnosis Point," press release, June 23, 1997.

20. D. Grady, "Fresh Guidelines Redefine Diabetes in Broader Terms," *New York Times,* June 24, 1997. Nathan goes on to say he supports the new guidelines, adding, "There is a cautionary side to this story."

21. Scandinavian Simvastatin Survival Study Group, "Randomized Trial of Cholesterol Lowering in 4444 Patients with Coronary Heart Disease: The Scandinavian Simvastatin Survival Study (4S)," *Lancet* 344 (1994):1383–89.

22. IMS America, "Top 10 Products—United States: Moving Annual Totals," Internet home page http://www.imsamerica.com:80/today/prod_sales.html. February 5, 1997.

23. T. S. Lesar et al., "Factors Related to Errors in Medication Prescribing," *JAMA* 277 (1977):312–17.

24. A. B. Witman et al., "How Do Patients Want Physicians to Handle Mistakes?" *Archives of Internal Medicine* 156 (1996):2565–69.

25. Thomas J. Moore, *Deadly Medicine* (New York: Simon & Schuster, 1995), chap. 16.

26. Pharmaceutical Research and Manufacturers of America, *Facts & Figures Backgrounders: Drug Safety* (see n. 19, chap. 3). Version reviewed November 16, 1996.

27. Ibid.

28. David C. Classen et al., "Adverse Drug Events in Hospitalized Patients," *JAMA* 277 (1997):301–6.

29. David W. Bates et al., "Incidence of Adverse Drug Events and Potential Adverse Drug Events," *JAMA* 274 (1995):29–34.

30. C. M. Lindley et al., "Inappropriate Medication Is a Major Cause of Adverse Drug Reactions in Elderly Patients," *Age and Ageing* 21 (1992):294–300.

31. Susanna E. Bedell et al., "Incidence and Characteristics of Preventable Iatrogenic Cardiac Arrests," *JAMA* 265 (199):2815–18.

32. Lucian L. Leape et al., "The Nature of Adverse Events in Hospitalized Patients," *New England Journal of Medicine* 324 (1991):377–84.

33. Judyann Bigby et al., "Assessing the Preventability of Emergency Hospital Admissions," *American Journal of Medicine* 83 (1987):1031–36.

34. Jane Porter and Hershel Jick, "Drug-Related Deaths Among Medical Inpatients," *JAMA* 237 (1977):879–81.

35. John F. Burnham, "Preventability of Adverse Drug Reactions," (Letter) *Annals of Internal Medicine* 85 (1976):80.

36. Goodman and Gilman, p. 1134. Other sources cite estimates from 1 in 10,000 to 1 in 60,000.

37. J. L. Sacks, "Bicycle-Associated Head Injuries and Deaths in the United States from 1984 Through 1988," *JAMA* 241 (1991):3016–18. Sacks reports that 87 percent of all bicycle-related head injuries resulted from collisions with automobiles.

38. Ibid.

13. GETTING THE FACTS

1. *Physicians' Desk Reference.*

2. Department of Health and Human Services, Food and Drug Administration, Advisory Committee on Antiviral Drugs, August 1994.

3. R. L. Fisher and S. Fisher, "Antidepressants for Children: Is Scientific Support Necessary?" *Journal of Nervous and Mental Disease* 184 (1996):99–108.

4. D. J. Kupfer, "Current Concepts: Management of Insomnia," *New England Journal of Medicine* 336 (1997):341–46.

5. United States Code of Federal Regulations, 21 CFR 201.57.

6. Ibid.

7. The FDA has created a dictionary of adverse reaction terms for its MedWatch system, but this is of little help to the consumer.

8. T. S. Lesar, "Factors Related to Errors in Medication Prescribing," *JAMA* 277 (1997):312–17. The study reported a rate of 3.99 errors per 1,000 prescriptions. But the hospitalized patient is typically prescribed between ten and twenty drugs during a typical stay.

INDEX